Children as Caregivers

The Rutgers Series in Childhood Studies

The Rutgers Series in Childhood Studies is dedicated to increasing our understanding of children and childhoods throughout the world, reflecting a perspective that highlights cultural dimensions of the human experience. The books in this series are intended for students, scholars, practitioners, and those who formulate policies that affect children's everyday lives and futures.

Edited by Myra Bluebond-Langner, Board of Governors Professor of Anthropology, Rutgers University, and True Colours Chair in Palliative Care for Children and Young People, University College London, Institute of Child Health

Advisory Board

Perri Klass, New York University

Jill Korbin, Case Western Reserve University

Bambi Schieffelin, New York University

Enid Schildkraut, American Museum of Natural History and Museum for African Art

For a list of all the titles in the series, please see the last page of the book.

Children as Caregivers

THE GLOBAL FIGHT AGAINST TUBERCULOSIS AND HIV IN ZAMBIA

Jean Hunleth

RUTGERS UNIVERSITY PRESS

NEW BRUNSWICK, CAMDEN, AND NEWARK, NEW JERSEY, AND LONDON

Library of Congress Cataloging-in-Publication Data

Names: Hunleth, Jean, 1976–author.

Title: Children as caregivers : the global fight against tuberculosis and HIV in Zambia / Jean Hunleth.

Other titles: Rutgers series in childhood studies.

Description: New Brunswick, New Jersey : Rutgers University Press, 2017. | Series: Rutgers series in childhood studies

Identifiers: LCCN 2016032166| ISBN 9780813588049 (hardcover : alk. paper) | ISBN 9780813588032 (pbk. : alk. paper) | ISBN 9780813588056 (e-book (epub)) | ISBN 9780813588063 (e-book (web pdf))

Subjects: LCSH: Child caregivers—Zambia. | AIDS (Disease)—Patients—Home care—Zambia. | HIV-positive persons—Home care—Zambia. | Tuberculosis—Patients—Home care—Zambia.

Classification: LCC HQ759.67 .H86 2017 | DDC 362.1096894—dc23

LC record available at https://lccn.loc.gov/2016032166

A British Cataloging-in-Publication record for this book is available from the British Library.

∞ The paper used in this publication meets the requirements of the American National Standard for Information Sciences—Permanence of Paper for Printed Library Materials, ANSI Z39.48–1992.

www.rutgersuniversitypress.org

Manufactured in the United States of America

For my parents, Frank and Mary Ann

Contents

Acknowledgments

Children as Caregivers is based on research I carried out in Lusaka during a time that spanned nearly ten years (2005, 2006, 2007 to 2008, and 2014). However, the ideas for the research took root much earlier when I was a Peace Corps volunteer in Eastern Province and then Central Province, Zambia (1999–2002). As a water sanitation volunteer in the village of Kapichila, near Lundazi, I was able to witness many things children accomplished for their families, and also the unacknowledged work that children put into global health projects. I thank Maxwell Banda and Anya Gondwe for opening their home to me and for putting their grandchildren in charge of introducing me to village life. Tikali, Regina, Suzgo, and Mattress taught me many lessons about children's creativity and the diversity of childhood experiences. I continue to carry these lessons throughout my career.

I have incurred many debts since starting the project that led to this book. I am beyond grateful for my longtime mentor, Karen Tranberg Hansen, whose deep knowledge of Africanist scholarship and her decades of research in Lusaka provided the foundation for my own work. Helen Schwartzman introduced me to the anthropology of childhood and pushed me to think creatively and critically about research with children. I thank both Karen and Helen for their unwavering support and the countless hours they have spent mentoring me through the years. I have benefited from the mentorship of so many other people, particularly Edward Fischer, Bill Leonard, Rebecca Wurtz, Caroline Bledsoe, Virginia Bond, Cathy Zimmerman, Brad Stoner, and Aimee James, who have all encouraged me, in different ways, to weave together my interests in anthropology and public health.

I have many people to thank in Zambia. My research affiliation with the Zambia AIDS Related Tuberculosis project (ZAMBART) proved vital, both when I was in Zambia and also back in the United States. Virginia Bond, in particular, assisted me in many ways, through pulling me into ZAMBART's projects, help-ing me seek research permissions, and being a wonderful interlocutor. Many other researchers and staff at ZAMBART, including Helen Ayles, Musonda Sim-winga, Mutale Chileshe Chibangula, Ab Schaap, and Levi Chilikwela, supported me along the way. The ZAMBART staff who worked in George, the site of my research—especially Angela Konayuma, Annie Mwale, Foster Chileshe, Violet Zulu, Janet Chisaila, Isaac Mshanga, and Faustina Moyo—deserve a big *zikomo* for their help and advice, and for enduring my presence in their small workspace at George Health Centre.

I am grateful for the assistance I received from the nurses and TB treatment supporters at George Health Centre. Floyd Makeka, a longtime TB treatment sup-porter, has been especially helpful, always encouraging my work and making me feel welcome, no matter how long my absences. Many other residents in George shared their homes and lives with me throughout the years and generously gave their time to this project, most especially the children and other household mem-bers who participated in my longest period of research during 2007 and 2008. I wish I could thank each of the participants by name, but the nature of this research has demanded that I use pseudonyms and change some identifying details to pro-tect their privacy. To acknowledge the time the children spent working with me, I have created an online gallery of the drawings they made as part of this research (see https://www.flickr.com/photos/childrenascaregivers/). It is the best way I know to follow eight-year-old Gift's advice: "Ba Jeanie, take my drawings to Amer-ica and show people how good my work is."

My research assistants, Emily Banda and Olivious Moono, worked so hard on this project and were exceptional guides into life in George. Emily had moved to George in 1964 as a young child. When we met, she was, and she continues to be, deeply committed to a number of development and faith-based projects focused on TB, HIV and AIDS, and orphans and vulnerable children. Olivious was twenty years old when we first met in 2007. After graduating from secondary school, she moved to George to live with family members and volunteer in HIV counseling and testing at the government health clinic. As I write this, she is finishing a nurs-ing degree. Both Emily and Olivious took on my research project as their own. The fact that they saw my study as worthwhile has meant more to me than any valida-tion I received through the years. Their tremendous efforts and their question-ing and critique of my research methodologies and assumptions make this book a shared accomplishment.

A number of friends in Zambia made my research possible through helping me with the logistics of traveling back and forth from the United States, and making Zambia feel like home each time I returned. Among these friends are Kelvyn Katongo, Steve Cole, Nsamwa Cole, Beth Jere, and Natalie Jackson. Ilse Mwansa, the former research affiliation officer at the Institute of Economic and Social Research at the University of Zambia, spent unhurried hours chatting with me about research and life and strongly encouraged me to finish this book. Wendy Nicodemus Constantinou and Chris Constantinou have cooked meals for me, lent me their car, set up housing for me, and shown me generosity beyond what I could ever expect.

This book would not have been possible without the funding and institutional support I received for the research and writing, particularly from a National Science Foundation Graduate Research Fellowship, a fieldwork grant from the Wenner-Gren Foundation for Anthropological Research, a fellowship from the Fulbright Institute for International Education, a writing fellowship from the American Association of University Women, and a number of small research grants from the Program of African Studies and Friends of Anthropology at Northwestern University. I previously published parts of chapter 4 in *Medical Anthropology Quarterly* 27, no. 2. Several passages were also published in *Childhood* and have been reproduced by permission of SAGE Publications Ltd., London, Los Angeles, New Delhi, Singapore, and Washington, DC, from "Beyond *On* or *With*: Questioning Power Dynamics and Knowledge Production in 'Child-Oriented' Research Methodology," *Childhood* 18, no. 1.

I appreciate all of the support I received to finish this book since arriving at Washington University's School of Medicine. I am especially grateful to Aimee James for believing in me, and this project, and for consistently encouraging me to finish. Graham Colditz, division chief of Public Health Sciences at Washington University, went out of his way to carve out a position that gave me the institutional support I needed to complete the book. I had the encouragement and support of many other colleagues: Rebecca Lobb, Natasan McCray, Meera Muthukrishnan, Julia Maki, Man-Yee (Mallory) Leung, Emily Benesh, Su-Hsin Chang, and Kathryn Henke. Grant Farmer, a brilliant epidemiologist and my co-conspirator in the Division, was a colleague who always got me. Grant touched so many lives, and he left this world before any of us were ready to say goodbye.

Many colleagues, friends, and family members have read and offered substantive comments on drafts of my book manuscript in its various forms: Karen Tranberg Hansen, Helen Schwartzman, Bill Leonard, Rebecca Wurtz, Virginia Bond, Mark Kent, Mary Ann Hunleth, Emily Steinmetz, Judith Singleton, Ana Croegaert, Olive Melissa Minor, Steve Cole, Joshua Garoon, Stephanie McClure, Priscilla Song, EA Quinn, and two anonymous reviewers for Rutgers University Press. Dawn Pankonien merits special mention for her critical comments at many stages of the writing, and especially after the sudden adoption of my newborn son. I thank Marlie Wasserman and Kimberly Guinta for all of the work they put into this manuscript and for their straightforward editorial advice that brought this book to fruition and made it stronger.

I am grateful to my family for their encouragement and insights, for the time they allowed me to work uninterrupted, and for pulling me away from my busyness with dinners, outings, and time spent together. One of the most profound moments I had during data analysis was with my niece, Alexa Hunleth, when she was three years old. Alex and I sat hunched over transcriptions of the children's interviews and storytelling sessions. I explained to Alex that I was finding important words in the transcripts. I asked her to find important words, too: pronouns. As she circled pronouns, I turned my attention to the pages in front of me to code for themes. When I looked back at Alex, I noticed that she had circled the word "love" in a number of places. After writing L-O-V-E at the bottom of a page, she told me, "Aunt Jean, there is a lot of love on the papers." I thank Alex for showing me the love in the children's stories and the necessity of incorporating love into my analysis.

I have so much love and gratitude for my parents, Frank and Mary Ann, who have always supported my unconventional approach to life and career and, in all of the most significant ways, made it possible. My husband, Mark Kent, has supported me, and the writing of this book, in too many ways to mention. This book was completed at a time of new beginnings for our family. As I worked through my revisions, Maxwell, our son, joined our family through adoption and renewed my energy to finish. Maxell, as tiny as he is now, has already expanded my view of family, care, and love beyond what I thought imaginable.

Children as Caregivers

Introduction

Maureen Nkhoma opened her eyes as I walked into her yard. Grabbing ahold of the well-worn quilt that covered her, she raised her head to acknowledge me. Her children, eight-year-old Loveness and twelve-year-old Bwalya, were hanging laundry nearby. She directed them to prepare the sitting room in their three-room house. "Outside is no good for a visit," she told me, as the wind swept dirt from the bare ground. It was a crisp August morning in Zambia's capital city, Lusaka.

"Get in," Maureen said, when she saw me hesitate at the door to her house. I had been watching her as she rose slowly on legs weakened from extended sickness and disuse. She walked toward the house with her gaze to the ground. Each uncertain step she took was filled with an effort that, I realized only later, she did not want me to see. At her insistence, I went into the sitting room ahead of her and took a seat across from Loveness and Bwalya. We sat in silence until Maureen joined us.

Maureen had tuberculosis (TB), a diagnosis that came after months of weight loss, fever, and night sweats, and a cough that had lingered for much too long. For the past thirty years, TB has ranked among the most pressing infectious diseases in the world, its presence and deadliness driven by political upheaval, public health neglect, poverty, and under-resourced healthcare systems, and made so much worse by the emergence of the HIV epidemic.[1] Globally, an estimated 9 million people become sick with and 1.5 million people die from the disease each year (UNOPS 2015).[2]

TB transcends national borders.[3] Globalization has increased the mobility of people, and complicated notions that TB—or any infectious disease—will remain confined to a particular nation or region. At the same time, TB offers a stark example of how global politics and policies have carved up the world in unequal ways, structuring who suffers from infectious diseases, who gets treatment, and who recovers.[4] Ninety-five percent of the deaths attributed to TB, for example, happen in middle- and low-income countries (World Health Organization 2015).

HIV and TB are an especially lethal combination in resource-poor areas. In Zambia, where Maureen Nkhoma lives, the incidence of TB rose dramatically in the 1980s, and in conjunction with the emergence and growing presence of HIV.[5] Debt to external lenders along with international policy reforms were gutting Zambia's healthcare system during the 1980s and 1990s, leaving the country unequipped to deal with the dual epidemic. TB medications ran short in Zambia during the latter part of the twentieth century. Antiretroviral therapy (ART) for HIV was unavailable to most people in the country until 2004, the year that ART was rolled out in government health clinics. People with HIV died ugly deaths, and these deaths were often the result of TB.[6]

Maureen's family was preparing for Maureen's funeral, her aging mother told me, when "everything changed." After months of undiagnosed illness, Maureen was hospitalized and tested positive for HIV. She was diagnosed with TB two weeks later, after her condition continued to decline while in the hospital.[7] In previous years, both diagnoses would have affirmed the family's concerns that Maureen would soon die. However, by 2007, the year that Maureen was diagnosed, medications for TB and HIV were widely available in Zambia at no cost to patients.

The new availability of no-cost medications for HIV and TB was not unique to Zambia. At the turn of the twenty-first century, significant global shifts in treatment policies, global markets, and funding streams were reconfiguring access to treatment around the world.[8] These shifts offered Maureen, like so many of her contemporaries in Zambia and elsewhere, hope for a "second chance at life" once diagnosed.[9] Second chances, though, are not a given in this new treatment-focused environment. As anthropologist Susan Reynolds Whyte has observed in the context of the rollout of ART in Uganda: "To realize the second chances, care must be given and taken continuously" (2014a, 2).

On the day that I visited Maureen and her children, Maureen did not yet know if she would have a second chance at life. She labored to reach the room where I waited with Loveness and Bwalya. When she finally arrived, she sank in exhaustion into the cushions of an overstuffed chair. After catching her breath, she glanced approvingly around the room. The walls were crumbling and couches threadbare. Yet, the concrete floor was swept and polished in a deep red. I noticed with embarrassment that the only traces of dirt were in the shapes of my own shoe prints. The tables were dust-free. Decorative cloths were freshly laundered and carefully draped over each couch cushion. I followed Maureen's gaze as she inspected each item in the room in turn, and then she turned to address me.

Connecting the condition of the room to the state of her care, Maureen said: "The children are taking good care of me. People would think it is the elders who are helping and cleaning the place, but it is the children." Maureen drew attention to the quality of her children's care. The children were not just taking care; they were taking good care of her. Their care was so good that people would think it was "the elders." The elders—her mother, brother, and other adult relatives—were not able to take such good care. They, too, had their own care needs and demands on their time. Months later, after Maureen completed more than eight months of TB treatment, she observed that her recovery from TB—her second chance at life, to use Whyte's phrase—was due, in large part, to her children's care.

A taken-for-granted assumption has shaped much global health research and policy work on infectious diseases around the world. This assumption is that adults, young or old, give care to the sick—an assumption that dismisses the many children who also give care to the sick. For example, millions of children in sub-Saharan Africa are estimated to provide some level of care as a result of the HIV epidemic.[10] More thoroughly discussed in the context of the HIV epidemic is the crisis of care that HIV has created for the children after their guardians have died.[11] The availability of treatment for HIV has helped raise life expectancy in heavily HIV-affected areas from what it had been before treatment. As a result, many children in sub-Saharan Africa and beyond now live with adults who benefit tremendously from medications, and yet face recurrent care needs.

Children as Caregivers takes the transition to and continued pursuit of universal treatment for TB and HIV as a critical moment in which to examine care between children and their ill family members. This book is set in a particular place, a poor urban settlement in Zambia, which has one of the highest rates of infectious disease in the country. The stories I tell in the following pages took place at a time (2005 to 2008, with follow-up research in 2014) when the delivery of health services to people with TB and HIV were changing many things about what it meant to receive such diagnoses. Yet residents were, and still are, grappling with the devastation the diseases wrought in their settlement during prior decades. Even with medications, deaths from TB and other HIV-related causes continue.

At its heart, *Children as Caregivers* is about how intergenerational care happens when infectious disease becomes woven into structures, relationships, and the rhythms of day-to-day life.[12] The argument I present throughout this book is that a focus on children's care for and by sick adults offers much-needed insight into global health problems and programs. This is no small argument; billions of dollars each year are invested in global health programming.[13] My argument has three interrelated themes. First, global processes, policies, and programs do not just affect children. They are also transformed by the intimate and everyday acts that occur between children and their family members.[14] In this respect, a study of care between children and their sick guardians can offer needed perspectives on larger political economic shifts, among these the increasing urbanization and feminization of poverty, brutal cuts to governmental healthcare spending, the uptick in magic-bullet approaches targeting specific diseases and groups, and the significant presence of non-state actors in the provision of services in middle- and low-income countries.

Second, a focus on relations between young children and ill persons offers important insight into the forms that care and sociality are taking within settings affected by high rates of infectious disease. Specifically, within recent infectious disease epidemics and outbreaks, target group categories such as orphan and vulnerable child, street child, and child-headed household have become the focus of media attention, humanitarian work, and academic research. By highlighting children's loss and isolation, such categories suggest that abandonment and isolation are what script children's lives. A focus on children's everyday interactions and relationships not only contextualizes their lives, but also honors the dependencies and interdependencies they cultivate and the meanings of such dependencies to their own and other peoples' lives.

Finally, children shape and are affected by global health, humanitarian, and medical programs, even when such programs are designed to exclude children. The global systems of public health and biomedicine are always contextualized pursuits, as Julie Livingston has shown in her study of cancer treatment in Botswana. Everywhere in the world, Livingston has reminded us, "doctors, patients, nurses, and relatives tailor biomedical knowledge and practices to suit their specific situations" (2012, 6). Part of seeing children as social actors is acknowledging that they, too, tailor global health, humanitarian, and biomedical systems of knowledge and practice to their particular circumstances, and as a means to make life more livable for themselves and other people. Understanding how they do so, I argue, is central to making policies accountable to children's circumstances and more relevant to their daily lives as well as the lives of their family and community members.

I have chosen to focus on TB, a disease that is overshadowed by HIV in social science research on children in sub-Saharan Africa. A study of TB in sub-Saharan Africa is in one sense a study of HIV, but from a different angle. While many illnesses and other ailments are viewed as signs of HIV's presence, TB strongly indexes HIV, even in the absence of a positive test result. With the increasing presence of ART, a biomedical TB diagnosis has also become the time when many people receive HIV diagnoses because of policies of direct HIV testing after TB diagnosis.

A study of TB offers much more than a lens onto the HIV epidemic. TB is the target of one of the farthest-reaching standardized global health interventions: the World Health Organization's (WHO) directly observed treatment, short-course (DOTS) strategy. DOTS has increased the availability of no-cost, outpatient TB treatment around the world and introduced a range of practices for monitoring treatment. Zambia reached 100 percent "DOTS coverage" in 2003 when all TB treatment programs run out of government health centers were based on the DOTS principles of testing, treatment, medication, observation, and reporting. The country's embrace of DOTS has precipitated a number of public-private partnerships aimed at treating the disease within the DOTS model.

Treatment coverage does not necessarily mean that medicines are accessible, nor should it imply that treatment adherence is an uncomplicated process of supplying drugs to the people who need them. As anthropologist Ian Harper (2006) has observed in Nepal, the DOTS protocol can feed into existing social hierarchies and be counterproductive to patient support. In this respect, attention to age and intergenerational relations offers a needed, and yet missing, perspective on DOTS in particular and standardized disease treatment protocols in general. A focus on children is especially compelling because TB has long been considered an "adult's disease," not only because of its association with HIV in sub-Saharan Africa, but also because of the difficulties in diagnosing TB in children. Children under fifteen years old account for only about 6 percent of the global burden.[15] Further distancing children, DOTS-based programs worldwide view caregivers as integral to TB treatment success, but these caregivers are assumed to be adults—an assumption that this book will soon dispel.

Children and the Practice of Being Closer

Throughout my research, I asked many questions and received many answers, but I have returned, in my thinking, to one particular question and its most common answer. I asked children living with adults who had TB: "How has this illness in your home changed your life?"[16] I posed a similar question to the adults with whom the children lived: "How has TB changed your child's life?" And child after child, adult after adult, offered me a similar response. The children made statements such as "I always wanted to be close to [my sick relative], now I want to *be closer.*" The children's parents, grandparents, and other sick guardians said: "The children always wanted to be close to me, but now they want to *be closer.*" At first I did not know what to make of these answers. "Being closer" seemed like a vague answer to my equally vague questions. Yet, I found the consistent references to proximity difficult to dismiss because of the infectiousness of TB. They were especially difficult to ignore when I witnessed children's attempts to stay close to relatives and the amount of effort entailed in sustaining such physical and emotional proximity.

The references people made to children's proximity hint at one of the central paradoxes of infectious disease: transmissibility creates conditions in which proximity is desired and necessary, and also feared. This is particularly true in settings where institutional and economic resources to treat infectious diseases are scarce. Relationships in such context are everything. Proximity can mark the quality of a relationship and serve as a critical strategy for social and biological survival, especially for people who are the most dependent upon others for their well-being. Let me offer an example to make this more concrete. On the day of Elesia's TB diagnosis, I sat in the house where she and her children, Abby and Chiko, were temporarily staying. Elesia was on the couch, next to several family members. Family members were discussing who in the family should care for Elesia and where they should send her children. Elesia stifled a series of coughs as she and her family worried about her six- and ten-year-old daughters' susceptibility to infection. Based on clinical advice about the infectiousness of TB and the rigorous eight-month treatment program, some family members suggested that it was best to separate Elesia from her children.

Over the course of two weeks, Elesia's sister gathered resources to move Elesia to her house on the other side of the city. Elesia's brother moved his wife and children to another relative's house to make room for Abby and Chiko in the house where he lived. Meanwhile, Abby and Chiko resisted the separation from their mother. They did so in specific verbal and nonverbal ways. They stayed closer to the house than they had before the family debate. They showed their ability to respond to their mother's physical needs, and they kept her company, prayed with her, and encouraged her to get better. They reflected on their futures without their mother and on the possibility of their mother's death while outside of their watchful care. There was no one who had more at stake in their mother's recovery than they did and this, they believed, made them most suitable to monitor her treatment and care. Elesia also wished to avoid the separation. However, by the time of the move, she was so sick that she had little energy to resist her family members' efforts.

When children spoke of wanting to be closer to specific persons, they were directing attention toward their relationships and dependencies as well as their strategies for cultivating interdependence. Their attempts to stay close evoked many of the ways in which anthropologists have studied care: as a form of work, as a sentiment and affective state, as an obligation and type of exchange, as an engagement with biomedicine, and as a process structured by social and economic inequality (Buch 2015, 279). Their care-based efforts to sustain relationships did not always work, as in Abby and Chiko's case, but children tried nonetheless, sometimes going to great extremes and, including, in the case of one young boy, running away from two different households in which he was placed.

Throughout this book, I examine the shared vulnerabilities of children and ill persons. I look most closely at how children attempted to minimize these vulnerabilities through cultivating relationships with specific ill guardians through acts of care. My intention is not to valorize this relationship between children and their sick relatives or downplay age-related inequalities and the scarcities that the children faced. Rather, I see the notion of "wanting to be closer" as a heuristic for examining children's social action. Since the 1970s, researchers in childhood studies have argued forcefully that we cannot understand children's lives without paying attention to children's own perspectives on their lives.[17] Their argument—an argument for which there is much proof—is that children interpret the world around them and act in ways that reproduce and also change this world. The attempt to remain close to particular ill persons, thus, represents one way in which children experienced and responded to illness and uncertainty, and also drew on the resources they had at hand—including the resources of biomedicine and the globalizing discourses of childhood—to craft particular approaches to care for themselves and other persons, in an attempt to maintain a sense of normality and retain hope for their futures.

How we define children's care for sick adults matters. Because children's caregiving was largely ignored by social scientists until rather recently, much research on children as caregivers has focused on the work of care, emphasizing children's domestic and nursing activities, their cooking, cleaning, nursing, bathing, feeding, and more. This positions children's care within the much larger body of research on children's domestic work,[18] which has made important contributions to our understandings of children's roles in economic life and shown that children's work can be quite significant in particular times and places.[19] A fundamental premise in childhood studies is that childhood is not a fixed life stage.[20] The cross-cultural variability in children's work exemplifies this premise. While there are universals shared by all young children around the world, such as small physical size and early dependence on persons older than them to meet their basic needs, there is much more variation in what children can and are expected to do. Furthermore, larger-scale processes—capitalism, urbanization, globalization, and, as I argue in this book, the changing apparatuses of global health—factor into what children do and also into ideologies about children's care work as normative and necessary, or out of place.

There is a tendency when examining children's work to want to identify it as good or bad, harmful or helpful. Children who carry out care work may be, in some cases, more vulnerable than children who do not, but this is not always the case. To draw a line between the acceptable and the harmful with regard to children's domestic work, international aid organizations and policy makers have relied on particular indicators, including age and amount of time spent engaged in domestic tasks. As anthropologist Rachel Bray (2003) has argued, such measures and, in fact, the international preoccupation with children's work above other aspects of their lives, can erase the contexts within which children's work is situated, thus hiding more than they reveal about children's insecurities and needs. Bray has offered the example of a young girl in South Africa. Responding to a survey on child labor, the girl gave answers that appeared to show that she did not engage in much domestic work at all. Her answers seemed like positive indicators of her well-being. However, when Bray went to the girl's home, she noticed that there were few chores for the girl to carry out because the household had almost nothing to clean or cook. In such a setting, Bray observed, a child's involvement in domestic work might actually be a positive gauge of social and economic security. In the example from my own study, Abby's and Chiko's inability to perform care work for their mother did not mitigate their vulnerability. Instead, it threatened their ability to influence the course of their mother's illness and, in their interpretation of events, their relationship with their mother and sense of security in the present and future. The point is that standardized measures only tell a partial, often decontextualized story, and this story does not always match children's experiences or their understandings.

Because children's contributions in households are highly variable, context specific, and do not map neatly onto age-based categories, the extent and nature of children's domestic work is hard to grasp. As anthropologist Pamela Reynolds (1991) has shown in her study of children's work in subsistence agriculture in Zimbabwe, one of Zambia's neighboring countries, anthropological research techniques are critical to understanding children's work in all of its complexity. Children's work, she suggested, can be at the same time obscured, not considered work, and also highly valued and valuable. It can also vary through time with the changing needs and capacities of households and children, making it hard to understand children's contributions at just one point in time. By following particular children through time, Reynolds was able to identify that children provided adjustable labor for households, filling in where needed and assisting other household members, typically women, when they were overburdened. Though Reynolds does not address illness, her points hold especially true in care for sick persons. The notion of being closer to the sick is far less vague if we think about care needs as constantly changing and if we consider staying close to an ill person as one way in which children remain knowledgeable of and able to do something about such health needs and changes.

Children's attempts to become even closer to specific guardians during illness were about much more than providing adjustable labor. As the example of Abby and Chiko demonstrates, the notion that children wanted to be closer also hints at another form of work—the work involved in retaining intergenerational and kin relationships. Anthropologist Fiona Ross (2010) has observed that the work of retaining social relationships is unending and frequently becomes most evident during crises, such as illness and death, when relationships threaten to dissolve and when social isolation and rejection become real possibilities. She has written about this work in terms of the temporality that illness and dying impose on ill persons: "Illness, death and talk of illness and dying insert new forms of time into daily routines and everyday life. Caring is pierced by waiting; plans are hollowed by uncertainties; time becomes rigid and drifts simultaneously. It is within and across these qualities of time and not solely those of chronology, seasonality and genealogy that social worlds are crafted and refashioned. The return to life involves . . . the crafting of relationships so that they again take a recognisable and socially sanctioned form" (2010, 198). While Ross was referring most specifically to adults who were ill, her observations are suggestive of the temporality that a guardian's illness might impose on children as well. As I will show throughout this book, children linked the survival of specific relatives to their own future prospects. Retaining closeness in proximity and affect served as a strategy to shape not only the social and biological survival of sick guardians, but also the social and biological survival of the child. This strategy was context specific and pulled from a range of discourses about proper relationships between children and adults and the types of relationships children need to attain livable futures.

Children's attention to their proximity to sick guardians highlights the broader inequalities that the children faced in their daily lives, as well as their attempts to do something about such inequalities. Anthropologist Frederick Klaits (2010) has offered insight on this point in his research in Botswana on how people were attempting to sustain relationships in the midst of the HIV epidemic. He suggested that broader economic inequalities in wage labor and access to resources had reinforced people's tendencies to assess the state of their relationships through the places in which they gave and received care. In Klaits's words, Batswana "have tended to experience social inequalities as aspects of gendered and generational relationships within domestic or housed spaces . . . As a result, they commonly take steps to reshape their own and other people's manner of imagining such relationships" (2010, 18). They did so through activities that occurred in households on a daily basis, such as bathing, nursing, drinking, visiting, and praying. While Klaits's observations were based primarily on women who were members of an Apostolic congregation, and not children, they resonate with the ways in which the children in my study worked to refashion their identities and relationships through activities that occurred between themselves and their sick guardians, in homes and on a daily basis.

Close attention to the place of care reveals both the inequalities children face and need to manage and also the increasingly global facets of childhood. Children received a range of messages about their schooling, rights, vulnerability, and work that they incorporated into their understandings of their situations and the care they gave and received (Skovdal and Ogutu 2009). These globalizing discourses of childhood, as I will argue throughout this book, cannot be measured against local discourses of childhood. They are localized in children's everyday lives. For example, the children in my study used categories, such as the category of the orphan, to interpret the social isolation that might occur if they were separated from a particular guardian. They understood their care work in particular places and for specific adults as a means of securing an education (and, thus, a future). They also construed activities carried out for the "wrong" adult as something that could inhibit their schooling. Abby, the girl I mentioned earlier who wished to stay with her mother to give her care, had been out of school since her mother became sick, but she saw her chances of returning to school as higher if she remained in her mother's care, rather than in her uncle's. In her mother's household, she was a caring daughter who responded to the needs of her mother. The potential for reciprocation remained there, despite her mother's debility. In her uncle's house, she saw herself as a domestic worker whose actions and attempts to develop a relationship and also receive resources went unreciprocated.

Research on children's experiences of caregiving frequently embraces dichotomous thinking: assessing children's care as negative or positive; seeing childhoods as local or global; and positioning children as caregivers or care receivers. This framework, I argue, limits our understandings of children's care. *Children as Caregivers* examines children's care in all of its complexity and "as many things all at the same time" (Orellana 2009, 118).[21] In the following chapters, I will show children's care for sick persons as a process of commensurability in which some children and ill adults forged—or attempted to forge—a common vulnerability, one in which boundaries between healthy and sick, adult and child became blurred.[22] It was this common vulnerability that the children and their ill guardians were referencing when they spoke of wanting and needing to remain close to one another.

Getting Closer

I wrote this book as an anthropologist who has worked for a number of years in the delivery of public health in Zambia, both prior to and during the research and writing of this book. I arrived in Zambia, first, as a Peace Corps volunteer and have since worked on a number of health assessments and interventions, with (or contracted by) the World Food Programme, UNICEF, and the Zambia AIDS Related Tuberculosis Project. Throughout this time, which spanned from 1999, when I joined Peace Corps, to my most recent anthropological fieldwork in 2014, I have seen how children's perspectives can become sidelined in the delivery of health services, even when services are aimed at children. I have also seen a growing emphasis on children's participation in public health interventions and community development, and I have struggled with my colleagues who work in the delivery of public health to identify ways to make children's participation in such processes meaningful.[23]

My interest in studying children's experiences with TB treatment and care grew out of my affiliation with a Lusaka-based nongovernmental organization, the Zambia AIDS Related TB Project, or ZAMBART.[24] Before beginning my own study of children's caregiving, I assisted ZAMBART staff with a project they were carrying out with schoolchildren. The project involved asking schoolchildren in heavily TB-affected settings to disseminate information about TB and HIV to their family members, with the hope that children might compel family members to get tested. It was the first TB project to involve children as health promoters in their communities, which made the project uniquely situated to answer a question that had never been asked: Do children have a role to play in TB prevention programming?[25] The children were already playing roles in their households, well beyond what the project envisioned. However, what exactly the children were doing in their households was hard to ascertain from their responses. We were missing the ethnographic details of children's daily lives with TB, and this raised further questions for me about what current and past public health efforts were also missing about the household management of the disease. This was a methodological problem that we could not solve within the confines of that project and certainly not within the many other studies of TB in Zambia and elsewhere that excluded children.

Much of what researchers know about people's experiences with TB comes from interview and survey-based studies, frequently carried out retrospectively and outside of the usual place of care, the home.[26] Such studies have identified important aspects of TB diagnosis and treatment, and yet they fail to adequately describe the range of social relationships that shape therapy management.[27] Instead, they hint at factors such as access to clinical resources, shortage of medications, and feelings of wellness that can only leave us to imagine the daily lives of TB sufferers and their household members. They frequently ignore children entirely. In the previous section, I demonstrated how statements about children's desires to stay close to ill persons helped me understand children's experiences and strategies in households affected by illness. The notion of being closer—or getting close—also offers an apt metaphor for ethnographic fieldwork.[28] Ethnographic fieldwork is about physical and social proximity: being in a particular place and close to particular people. Ethnographers live, work, or visit with people repeatedly over time. Observation and participation in daily life brings researchers closer to people's daily lives and relationships than other social science and community-based methodologies, which tend to rely on a limited number of interactions conducted outside of the usual places where people live, work, receive care, and generally carry out their daily activities.

The Research

Because I wanted a closer perspective on daily life with TB, I chose to situate most of my research in the clinic and in houses in one particular place—George—a poor residential area that is located on the geographic and economic margins of Lusaka. Lusaka is both the capital of Zambia and the largest city in the country, with around 2 million residents in 2015, in a country of more than 15 million people. Approximately 70 percent of Lusaka's residents live on just 20 percent of the city's land, in low-income areas that encircle the city (World Bank 2002). George is one of these settlements. Through various exclusions, residents of George face high risks of infectious diseases such as TB. It has been estimated that the incidence of active TB in George is 800 in every 100,000 individuals per year (UNICEF 2008), a number nearly double the country-level incidence.

George is a favored location for international nongovernmental organizations (NGOs) and research for several reasons. The health statistics in the area provide the methodological as well as moral and practical justifications that researchers and practitioners need to show funders. There is an infrastructure for and history of health projects at the government health center in George. There is also a clear need to improve and provide services that are sorely lacking. The first time I went to George was in 2005 with my colleagues at ZAMBART, who were working with the government health center to carry out research on TB diagnostic testing and promote TB reduction initiatives.[29] Since that first visit, I have carried out my own fieldwork in the settlement in 2005, 2006, 2007 to 2008, and 2014, with the help of two research assistants who lived in George, Emily Banda and Olivious Moono.

The central observations in this book come from twenty-five households, each of which I visited weekly during my 2007 to 2008 fieldwork, and then again in 2014.[30] Of these households, seventeen households had an adult member (eight women and nine men) who had been diagnosed with active TB at the initiation of my research. Eight households were comparison households, households in which no one had been diagnosed with TB for the previous five years.[31] Because I was interested in examining children's care, I focused most directly on children between the ages of eight and twelve years old. All twenty-five households had at least one child in this age range, for a total of thirty-eight children (twenty girls and eighteen boys). I chose this age group because children of this age are so frequently left out of global health and medical research, which has focused primarily on children under age five years and fifteen years and older. In addition to the observations, interviews, and other methods I carried out in these twenty-five households, I also administered a broader survey across two hundred households in George, carried out observations in clinical sites of TB treatment, and conducted participatory workshops with children.[32]

One of the many things I find so valuable about ethnographic research and writing is the ability to combine many different forms of evidence, from observations made while participating in activities of daily life to interviews, structured surveys, performances, archival materials, and much more. I find such an approach not only necessary for examining health and illness, but also critical to understanding children's experiences and perspectives. In recent years, much has been written about the best ways to include children in research, with many debates and discussions about the value of various, usually participatory techniques.[33] As will become evident throughout this book, I relied on many techniques for working with children, including observations in their households as well as more participatory approaches, such as performance, group discussions, games, and drawing. (View the children's drawings at https://www.flickr.com/photos/childrenascaregivers/.) Flexibility, variability, and constant reflection defined my approach to research with the children. My analysis does not privilege any one method. I draw on all of the methods I used to bring me closer to understanding children's strategies for and perspectives on care.

Ethnography and Illness

Ethnographic research aims to humanize people, but infectious diseases can be dehumanizing. Airborne diseases such as TB produce fears—both real and imagined, with the lines often blurring between the two. Many people over the years have asked me if I was worried that I would contract TB. I was concerned for myself and also for Emily and Olivious and the people we might expose if we became sick. We took precautions, but there were also limits.[34] Complete avoidance would have meant shunning the things that humanize people during illness, such as sitting quietly together or entering a bedroom to offer words of encouragement to a person who could not get out of bed. People made counter attempts to avoid transmitting TB to us. They stifled coughs and made sure that we sat near doors that were opened wider than usual to let air circulate. We paid attention to these signs and adjusted our behavior. Paying attention to proximity—and also limiting our proximity—served to build the relationships that were essential to this research.

Tuberculosis, like most serious diseases, creates crises in households that shape the research relationship, particularly during initial diagnosis and at times when symptoms are severe.[35] Another question that I receive frequently is: How much did I intervene in or help the households in my study? This question comes particularly from students and practitioners of medicine and public health who are new to ethnographic research and worry about the ethical implications of observing suffering. I have two responses. The first is that I did provide some assistance. Emily, Olivious, and I put people in touch with various aid programs that gave monthly allocations of food and other resources. The three of us were frequently asked for biomedical information. Emily and Olivious gave advice based on their previous work with HIV- and TB-related programming, and we contacted doctors and TB nurses to field questions we could not answer. I sometimes gave money for transportation to health centers or the University Teaching Hospital, or for follow-up X-rays or diagnostics tests. I brought nutritious foods to households when it seemed that there was not enough food in the house. While I have no illusion that I was more than a blip in people's lives, I acknowledge that my presence shaped illness management and illness trajectories and, therefore, the research in ways that I will never fully know.

My second answer to this question addresses a broader concern, especially for people with previous experience working in or studying medicine, public health, and social work who are accustomed to interventions. I reiterate the value of slowing down in a global public health research environment that values action, speed, and efficiency.[36] This slowing down forefronts listening first and not assuming that we know what is best for people in different circumstances from us. In teaching interview techniques in health research, I have learned that many people unfamiliar with ethnographic interviewing are inclined toward correcting or judging people who say things that fall outside of the parameters of biomedicine, taking an expert stance that positions them as knowledge producers. This contradicts a fundamental aspect of ethnography in which informants are the knowers and the ethnographer is the person striving to know (Madison 2012). I teach that the benefits of listening and taking a nonexpert position are many. Such a position enables us to learn how things work on the ground and to get past our taken-for-granted assumptions about people's lives. It allows us to question received ways of categorizing people and problems and intervening in people's lives. That is, listening to people and seeing issues from multiple perspectives can offer more appropriate pathways for changing the delivery of healthcare and medicine (Biehl and Petryna 2013a; Pigg 2013).

OVERVIEW OF THE BOOK

Each chapter in *Children as Caregivers* engages children's perspectives on their circumstances, while addressing a different aspect of the children's daily lives. The chapters progressively build to develop a fuller understanding of the children's caregiving within a setting heavily affected by infectious disease. The first chapter, "Growing Up in George," situates the reader in the urban residential area where the children lived, describing the many factors, including global restructuring and a history of international development agendas, that have shaped the landscape and children's life chances. The children's perspectives on this landscape offer lessons applicable to the growing array of global health efforts in poor, urban environments around the world.

In chapter 2, "Residence and Relationships," I move my analysis into the domestic sphere and examine children's changing roles in and across households in the HIV era. Family has become a critical concept in global endeavors to assist children in settings affected by infectious disease. Many observers have identified the limits to families' abilities to care for children in places with high burdens of adult illness and death. The notion of children "in family care" as opposed to "outside of family care," on the streets or in institutions, has gained particular traction in international attempts to provide resources to children. Despite the explicit attention given to the notion of family in research and program development in HIV-affected areas, children's roles as family members have not been adequately conceptualized. This chapter focuses on the active ways in which children were shaping family networks and attempting to cultivate relationships with particular people in order to receive good care.

Caring for children can be particularly challenging during illness and, in many places in Africa and around the world, aspects of TB and HIV diagnoses can exacerbate these challenges. Chapter 3, "Between Silence and Disclosure," explores the issue of disease disclosure to children, starting with the observation that most adults in my study did not disclose their TB diagnoses to their children. Increasingly, public health research seeks answers to why adults do or do not disclose disease diagnoses to children, and the effects of disclosure on children's present and future well-being. I suggest that this line of investigation, which focuses on what is not said, obscures the many ways of knowing and communicating about illness. This chapter calls for an extreme broadening of definitions of disclosure to include the silent presences of disease and acknowledge the relationship-building practices that occur in the absence of a named disease. I make an even broader point about how we theorize children's and adult's agency within infectious disease epidemics, and how this has ramifications on global health programming and research.

Chapter 4, "Following the Medicine," continues to show children's active involvement during illness through describing their participation in and responses to changing TB control measures in Zambia. In the twenty-first century, TB drugs have become increasingly available and regulated by a range of international donors and actors, and in compliance with the World Health Organization's DOTS strategy. Even though the children were rarely allowed at the clinical site of TB treatment in George, they viewed their actions outside of this site as integral to TB treatment adherence. They appropriated the global discourses of TB treatment and used these to attain belonging and make claims to households. Children's uses of the materials and discourses of TB treatment offer a strong case for the value of children's perspectives on global health technologies, even when such technologies are not aimed at children.

TB treatment has not been a magic bullet. Poverty, an overburdened healthcare system, and many other factors prolong and worsen suffering from the disease in George and other heavily TB-affected areas in sub-Saharan Africa. Families assume much of the expense as well as the work of caring for people with TB, just as they have for other debilities and diseases. Within families, however, the expense and work of caring is not distributed equally, and women in particular, in all parts of the world, face the highest caregiving loads. The social and economic inequalities that shape women's burdens of care work also make women more vulnerable to infectious diseases, including TB. Chapter 5, "Care by Women and Children," provides an in-depth view of two women's illness trajectories. In both cases, there was a seeming absence of adult kin involvement in the women's care. Children filled this void. This chapter underscores the significance of gender and age-related inequalities, while also showing how women and children attempted, through proximity to one another, to minimize the disruptions to their present and future well-being. Chapter 5 reaffirms a common theme throughout the book: social relationships shape the kinds of care people get, and children must be viewed as part of—rather than at the margins of—caregiving relationships.

I continue to draw out the importance of including children's caregiving actions and relationships in my conclusion, "Children and Global Health," as I tie together the central lessons from the book. This concluding chapter shows the immediate and dire need for far more complex understandings of children and childhoods than those presently held within the field and practice of global health. In both this concluding chapter and a postscript on recent efforts to treat childhood TB, I offer lessons and questions as funding and programs increasingly turn their attention to children.

A Note on Writing

Children's views are the central focus of *Children as Caregivers*. I have attempted to remain true to the accounts that the children offered, while acknowledging that I have filtered their words and experiences through my own interdisciplinary lenses (those of anthropology, childhood studies, and public health). I wrote this book with several distinct audiences in mind, among these: students and other people interested in global health disparities, practitioners working in disease control or with child welfare programs, anthropologists who focus on illness and caregiving, and childhood researchers from various disciplines. In writing for different audiences, I agonized over word choices and wondered how my descriptions brought me closer to or farther away from the terms the children used to describe their experiences. I discovered, as Barrie Thorne has written, "that different angles of vision lurk within seemingly simple choices of language" (1993, 8). Because of this, I wish to make explicit some of my language choices and challenges.[37]

In both scholarship and policy documents on children living in adversity, children are frequently labeled or categorized according to particular circumstances or needs. These are cultural constructions, as I will show throughout this book. They hold specific purposes in policy and research: to account for need, bring attention to a particular social issue, or study the extent of a problem. Common labels used within the HIV epidemic are orphan and street child. The labels *child carer* and *child caregiver* are also entering into the vocabulary of researchers and practitioners to indicate children who care for people who are sick, debilitated, and elderly, or for younger children. Most children I knew in George would not categorize themselves in these ways, or they would use such labels only very selectively. Because of this, I have tried to limit categorizing the children by labels except in cases in which the children used them or I directly discuss literature and programs aimed at a specific category of children. Avoiding such terminology removed the limitations I had in my own thinking, particularly on what care and family might look like. It enabled me to identify many aspects of care that I had previously not considered and also see the interdependence in children's actions and sentiments.

I struggled, too, with the language I used to write about TB and HIV. Most public health and medical research makes disease diagnosis an explicit part of study participants' identities. In certain ways, my work is no different because of my focus on people diagnosed with TB. However, I have not focused solely on these diseases and I have purposely left some diagnoses unwritten. As I will show, HIV and TB were not named so directly in many of my conversations, and many guardians and their children actively resisted having their lives reduced to diagnoses, preferring to fashion themselves in other ways, as, for example, mothers, fathers, daughters, sons, or grandparents. TB and HIV were ever-present in family life, and yet there was much more to children's lives and relationships than the TB or HIV diagnosis, which I show throughout this book.

A main goal of the book is to offer the details and context that are so frequently missing in reports and articles on infectious disease prevention and on childhoods in adversity, as well as to provide new frameworks for viewing illness, treatment, childhood, and family. My account focuses specifically on children's lives at one place and time to make real for the reader the hardships children face while also showing how children create relationships, make do, and give meaning to life within such constraint. I have worked to show readers the value of ethnographic research and writing for understanding these challenges as well as honoring children's creative responses to adversity. I have also worked to show ethnographers of global health the value of including children in their analyses. I hope that my work will make readers question the status quo in global health research and practice concerning children. I hope, too, that my work will introduce some avenues for change in global health programming and policies and that children, in particular, will experience such changes as beneficial.

CHAPTER 1

Growing Up in George

In a fascinating cartographic depiction, nine-year-old Luka Kangwa drew for me the shape of Zambia in abstract likeness to official representations of the country. Using red, green, brown, and black crayons, Luka marked off Zambia on an otherwise colorless page, dividing the country into five sections to represent its different provinces.[1] He drew a small circle with three lines extending below the country. The line on the right extended down, becoming two parallel lines that meandered across the page, eventually ending at the door of a small house. This, he told me, was the house in which he lived with his mother, father, eleven-year-old brother, and older sisters. A larger, more prominent, pencil-darkened road extended out of the Zambian map, leading downward and branching off. To the left, Luka had drawn a gathering of stick people and stick tables. "This is the market," he said, "where I am sent to buy things." The branch on the right curved slightly and extended down to a large, detailed football field where Luka drew himself playing a game of football with his friends. The places on Luka's map were predictable: the football field (located within his school grounds), home, and market.

I read Luka's map in three ways. In one reading, his map reveals a distinctly local experience of childhood. In another reading, we can see the familiarity of the places he identified (home, school, football field, market) to many children around the world. These places are global structures. And in yet another reading, Luka's creative placement of his everyday world within a larger nationalistic space demonstrates the interconnectedness of the local and global. The places he went were neither bounded nor unaffected by larger processes, including global processes, yet they were also not determined by such processes. He showed himself on the map, playing on the field and buying in the market, and he placed himself strategically at the juncture between the map of Zambia and the roadways.

Children in George live in a global world, and they experience global structures and globalizing discourses of childhood, just as do children around the
world (James and James 2012). This chapter examines the particular ways in
which children were experiencing growing up in George, one of many poor
urban settlements in Zambia. Social disadvantage is experienced in spatial terms
in Lusaka, as it is in many cities (Beall 2002; Hansen 2005). Lusaka's poor residents often do not have the networks, schooling, or certificates to attain jobs
in service and high-tech businesses, or in the growing number of international
nongovernmental organizations. High-end malls and restaurants are nearby, but
the products they sell are too expensive for the poor. Families get stuck in the
low-income housing areas that encircle the city, with the labor markets of globalization further marginalizing them. And yet, the urban poor in Lusaka live in a
global world. Like members of the middle and upper classes in Lusaka, they tune
in to movies, television shows, and soap operas set in more affluent locales of
Africa and around the world. They are exposed to the discourses of international
organizations regarding their rights about housing, schooling, work, and health.
In effect, the processes of globalization simultaneously exclude and include the
urban poor, including children (Hansen 2005).

Children living in poor urban areas have little control over the macro processes that shape the places where they live. Nevertheless, they are neither passive victims nor simply observers of these processes.[2] Given the millions of
children living in urban poverty around the world, this is not just a chapter
on a particular settlement in Lusaka, but one that addresses the importance
of understanding how children perceive their lives and the environments in
which they grow up. Children's perspectives, I argue, can offer insight into the
design of health and development programs and policies. At present, many
such efforts misconstrue children's lives and livelihood strategies and misun-
derstand how children engage with global development discourses. My intention, therefore, is to show how global health and development programs might
draw on both the contexts of children's lives and also children's perspectives to
better inform their agendas.

I begin this chapter with an overview of the history of George, starting when
the land was first developed into a peri-urban residential area on the outskirts
of Lusaka.[3] While the details of George's development are unique, the story
should sound familiar to readers working in other peri-urban areas in Africa
and beyond. Taking my cue from Luka and the other children who mapped
their surroundings for me, I have chosen to describe four aspects of George
in depth in this chapter: housing and home ownership; international development projects, represented by a standpipe water (*kajima*) system; schooling;
and global public health education initiatives.

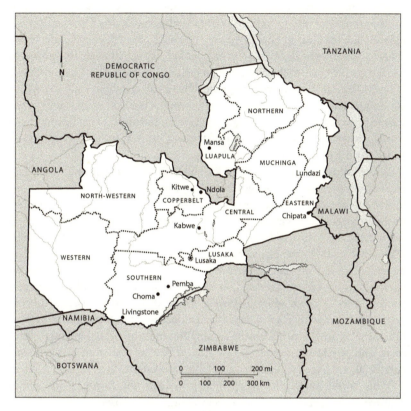

Fig. 1.1 Map of Zambia, 2016.

From Farmland to Poor Urban Settlement

George's development as a residential area began in the 1960s. At that time, Zambia was the symbol of an "emerging Africa"; the nation was urbanized and urbanizing (Ferguson 1999). Zambia was and still is a major exporter of copper, with copper mining driving the country's economy. Just after Zambia's independence from Britain in 1964, Zambia had one of the highest per capita incomes in Africa and was considered a middle-income country. In the 1960s and early 1970s, employment opportunities were aplenty in Lusaka, attracting many people, and their families, to a city that was not designed for a large population. The farms on the outskirts of town were the main space where the new residents could settle.

George provides one example of peripheral rural area turned residential settlement.[4] The settlement received its name from a man named George, an *azungu* (foreigner) rumored to be from either Britain or Greece, depending upon whom you ask. George or Haji George (again, depending on whether the speaker considers him to be British or Greek) occupied the farmland prior to 1964. He left the land and his farmhouse when Zambia became an independent country. Some say he fled back to Britain. Others say he remained in Zambia, but handed the land over to the new government and opened a guesthouse elsewhere in town. Regardless of where George went, his small farmhouse still stands. Age has disintegrated its bricks and concrete flooring. A bare, dirt yard stands in contrast to the colorful gardens I imagine once surrounded the house. George's view was expansive. The house now looks on to many other houses, as neighbors have closed in on it through the decades.

While farms provided open land for building, their physical and social marginalization presented challenges to their new urban residents.[5] Transportation to the city center from the outer-lying farms was difficult. Because the land was not recognized as part of the city, residents had minimal access to city services, including basic amenities such as clinics, schools, trash collection, streetlights, and roads. By the 1970s, the government acknowledged the considerable investments residents had made in these lands. They also recognized the lack of resources available to residents, who endured poor living conditions that fostered poverty (Hansen 1997). Beyond Zambia, there was widespread international concern about urban slums. International agencies turned their attention to improving such areas, with the assumption that substantial attention to the social and physical infrastructure in these areas was needed to prevent health and social problems for residents, and for entire nations.

With World Bank funding from 1976 to 1980, the Zambian government endeavored to upgrade the conditions in George and incorporate it into the city. Upgrading plans included resettlement and rebuilding of housing, construction of roads, installation of streetlights, and provision of trash collection and other services. These plans, however, were fraught with problems, including financial problems brought on by the global oil crisis in 1973 and the decline in demand for copper on the global market in the first half of the 1970s.[6] By the official end of upgrading in 1982, architect and longtime researcher in George, Ann Schlyter, observed: "garbage collection had been organized, [but] it was not efficient, street lighting was not provided, the schools did not cover needs, no clinic was provided, standpipes run short of water, and some of the roads needed maintenance" (1984, 47).

The global financial crisis not only halted Zambia's realization of improved low-income residential areas; it dramatically changed the lives of urban dwellers in general. Because of the crisis, the government had to borrow extensively from external lenders, principally the International Monetary Fund (IMF) and the World Bank (WB), to support the country. From 1970 to 1990, Zambia's external debt rose from US$ 627 million to US$ 7.2 billion (Rakner 2003). This debt came with strings attached, including the implementation of structural adjustment programs in the 1980s and 1990s and a shift to a market-based economy in the 1990s. Although intended to spur economic growth, these policies amounted to an assault on public sector programs and spending. Increased privatization and the scaling back of the public sector proved to have detrimental effects on people's health and well-being, which have been documented widely for Zambia and other countries (Pfeiffer 2013).

Statistics in urban Zambia convey part of the story of human suffering associated with the policy shifts in the late twentieth century. During the 1990s, urban residents in Zambia became even poorer than they were in the late 1970s, and urban poverty reached nearly 50 percent in 1994 (Ferguson 1999). Residents of George experienced the economic downturn and donor-imposed reforms in specific ways: a shortage of jobs, overcrowding and a lack of access to adequate housing, the elimination of state subsidies for food and transportation, and the loss of entitlements for healthcare and education. They also experienced reforms as hunger and an increase in infectious diseases such as TB, HIV and AIDS, and cholera. With conditions worsening and limited national and international help, residents described feeling abandoned by their government and the international community.

Recognizing the detrimental effects of structural adjustment programs, global advocacy groups developed campaigns in the 1990s to push international funding institutions to forgive national debts and focus instead on poverty reduction. In 2000, Zambia entered the Heavily Indebted Poor Countries initiative, a program aimed to relieve the massive debt that countries accumulated during the preceding years. The country completed the program in 2005 and received US$ 3.8 billion in debt relief. As a condition for debt relief, Zambia and other countries had to prepare poverty reduction strategy papers (PRSPs), documents meant to direct debt relief into developing poverty-focused government programs and increase spending in key areas such as gender equality, health, and education. Despite the explicit focus on poverty reduction, however, critics have suggested that the PRSPs are merely a euphemism for the structural adjustment programs of earlier years. The same neoliberal ideology informs the PRSPs, with continued reliance on privatization and the scaling back of the public sector (Pfeiffer 2013).

Even though Zambia continues to have very poor health indicators, and George has among the worst health indicators in the country, the twenty-first century has brought numerous changes. The United Nation's Millennium Development Goals laid out a set of global benchmarks that gave concrete health, educational, and other targets for countries to work toward. New global health players entered the development scene. These include the Bill and Melinda Gates Foundation, the US President's Emergency Plan for AIDS

Relief, pharmaceutical companies, and research initiatives.[7] This global presence is revealed in projects that offer services that the government cannot provide, including, as we will see in later sections, the provision of basic needs such as water, health services, and schooling.

The land that makes up George is no longer farmland; it is part of Lusaka's densely populated urban sprawl. In 2005, best estimates suggested that 117,825 people lived in the residential area.[8] As of this writing, it is likely that the population is closer to 130,000. George is now a well-connected urban settlement, where residents come from all parts of the country. I administered a questionnaire in 200 households in George that captured some of the ethnic diversity and complex migration histories of residents. Twenty-four percent of heads of households were born in George, 28 percent came to George from another residential area in Lusaka, 17 percent moved from Eastern Province, 15 percent from Copperbelt Province, and 5 percent from Central Province. Smaller numbers of people moved to George from each of the other provinces in Zambia and also South Africa and Zimbabwe. The earliest recorded move to George was in 1959 and the latest in 2008, just weeks prior to the survey.

George can feel small and even familiar, and it can also feel large and divided. Residents rarely refer to themselves as being from George. Instead, they list many formally and informally named areas in the settlement, such as Lilanda, Down Kawama, or George Proper. The dividedness of George was brought home to me late one afternoon while I sat with my research assistant, Emily, and we thumbed through a stack of household surveys Emily had completed. Each one of the surveys had the same surname written across the front. "Emily," I asked, "how did you manage to interview only Bandas today?" Five households with the same surname along a preselected transect seemed improbable, even if Banda was a common name in Eastern Province, Zambia. That they shared a surname with Emily made it even more incredible. She joked, "I feel good today because I spent the day with my brothers and sisters." I asked if she knew them. She did not, but they looked familiar. Then she explained something quite simple: when people move to George from the village, they try to live near relatives, creating clusters of households with similar ethnic backgrounds and, sometimes, shared surnames.

Despite the many residential groupings, people of different ethnicities and backgrounds can live next door to one another without discord. In fact, the insecurity of the rental housing market in recent years has meant that renters do not have much choice about exactly where they live or for how long. Neighbors will speak to one another in Lusaka Nyanja or Lusaka Bemba, locally used terms

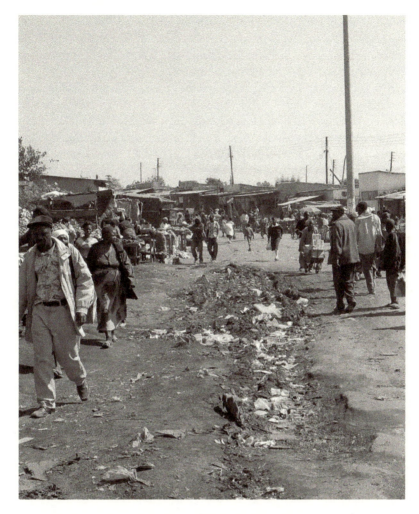

Fig. 1.2 The largest market in George and the main road to the government health center during the 2008 rainy season. Photo by Rosha Forman.

for the two most common language varieties spoken in the capital city. Like the Town Bemba described by linguistic anthropologist Deborah Spitulnik, Lusaka Nyanja and Bemba are fluid and creative languages that represent the "hetero-geneous nature of urban life" (Spitulnik 1998, 33). These language varieties are strongly intertwined with ideas of modern urban as opposed to traditional rural life. Lusaka Nyanja and Lusaka Bemba provide ways for people to communicate when they do not share the same native language, and they serve as the first languages of most children born in George. Other native languages (there are around fifteen to twenty distinct languages and many more dialects) as well as deep forms of Nyanja and Bemba are hardly dismissed in everyday interactions. Instead, these languages promote lively conversation and are seen as purer forms of language associated with traditional rural living.

With the growth of the settlement and the increasing presence of newcomers, residents must find ways to respond to linguistic and ethnic diversity. Because of the two years I spent as a Peace Corps volunteer in Lundazi, people I met reframed me as a Tumbuka, an honorary they used to position me closer to them than I was as a person from the United States. I was regularly asked to teach people Tumbuka phrases when they found out about my background. It was surprising to hear a white woman speak Tumbuka, particularly because the region of Zambia where people speak Tumbuka is far from Lusaka. But rather than teasing me about my pronunciation or seeing my language abilities as a novelty, they took my knowledge seriously, repeating my phrases. When newcomers arrived from Tumbuka-speaking areas of the country, I was asked to speak Tumbuka with them. This was not to make me comfortable, but to put the newcomers at ease. In a similar way, my research assistant, Olivious, was asked questions about Tonga and called to talk with people arriving from Southern Province.

The conversations about languages in which people engaged on a daily basis were not trivial. They accomplished serious work when people met for the first time or when newcomers arrived from distant places. Such acknowledgment served as an effort—whether it was conscious or unconscious—to use language differences and similarities to strengthen ties among diverse people. It tied in with larger political efforts in Zambia to value ethnic diversity and, at the same time, promote unity under the national motto: "One Zambia, One Nation."

Despite a measured wariness of outsiders, residents treated newcomers with generosity, particularly when they viewed the newcomers as even worse off than they, the residents, were. In 2008, there were a number of Zimbabwean women who had traveled to Lusaka and ended up in George. Zimbabwe, the country just south of Zambia, was experiencing a prolonged period of hyperinflation during that time, which ultimately led the country's leaders to abandon their currency. The selling of goods in Zimbabwe was precarious because the free fall of the Zimbabwean dollar meant that all money collected lost its value immediately. Struggling to survive, some market women from Zimbabwe made their way across the border and up to Lusaka to sell prepackaged biscuits. No one could tell me how or why they came to George to sell their biscuits, but their presence prompted commentary on how hard life was for women in Zimbabwe. Emily, Olivious, and other women I knew made a special point to buy the biscuits sold by these women, reminding me how small actions between people produce civility in harsh socioeconomic and environmental conditions.

How Children Described George

Several months after the start of my research in 2007, I sat in the office of the regional security officer at the US Embassy, awaiting a security briefing. I was beginning a yearlong Fulbright Fellowship for which it was his job to ensure my safety. He asked about the location of my apartment. I lived in Kabulonga, a high-income area of the city. He approved, though he questioned the number of locks, exits, and burglar bars, and whether or not the wall fence was high enough and the wires on top sufficiently electrified. He arranged for a US marine to investigate these issues further. He warned me about safety around town. I should proceed with caution in the city center. I should not take taxis or mini-buses. And I should never—never ever—venture into the *compounds*. In the language used to classify space in Lusaka, George is a *compound*. I thanked the regional security officer for the warning and let him know that I planned to drive to George Compound after we spoke.

In the colonial era, the term *compound* had a very specific meaning. It referred to the racially segregated housing areas set aside for African workers to build their own houses or live in housing provided by employers.[9] The term was contrasted with the term *mayadi*, which comes from the English word "yard," and was used during the colonial era to refer to white residential areas.

Despite the end of colonial rule, the designation between compound and mayadi persists. The distinction is now structured by income rather than race. Compound has come to stand for all low-income neighborhoods in Lusaka. Mayadi stands for high-income neighborhoods, but people living outside of the compounds rarely use this descriptor and many foreign aid workers I knew were unfamiliar with the word. Power inequalities are evident in the differential usage and knowledge of these descriptors. For example, compound serves as an adjective that modifies a placename, such as George Compound. However, mayadi does not. I lived in Kabulonga, not Kabulonga Mayadi.

In its current usage, the term compound is encoded with a number of meanings. The regional security officer invoked the term to imply criminal activity and danger posed to US workers abroad who venture outside of designated safe spaces. My friends at international NGOs use it differently to talk about need and development aid in Lusaka. The compounds are where many global projects are set. Compound tours exist to show visitors to Zambia the poverty in the country. I knew a woman in George whose foreign-funded church tasked her with taking European visitors around George in the hopes that they would give generously to support the church's activities. After each visit, she expressed to me her disappointment that the visitors looked upon the residents of George with pity, and yet they never tried to talk with them and frequently left without a donation. It made her feel like George was a spectacle.

Negative connotations of compounds abound, just as they do for townships, slums, squatter settlements, and ghettos in other parts of the world. I was interested in learning how children described compounds and their residence in such places, and so, during a group discussion with the children, I asked them to describe the difference between compound and mayadi. Here are some of their answers:

GIFT: Like in Woodlands [a high-income area] there are no careless children like we have careless children here.

OLIVIOUS: In what way are they careless?

MARY: There [in mayadi], they are clean. If you tell children to throw *nshima* [the staple food in Zambia], they will throw it in the bin, while children in the compound will throw anywhere.

MULENGA: If you tell a child in the compound to throw nshima in the bin, he will just throw it by the doorstep.

GRACE: It's better living there than here because of mud houses with no electricity [here], while good residential areas have nice houses with wall fences, painted walls, showers, flushing toilets.

ABBY: In George, there are ugly houses.

AGNES: Houses made of mud—

SAMSON: —with grass on top.

MUSA: In mayadi they [the people] are clean unlike here where they are dirty. In mayadi [people] are not illiterate.

AGNES: The people in mayadi look clean, not like here. Here in some houses there are even rats.

These quotes make evident how quick the children were to point out the negative connotations and judgments encoded in the term compound when compared with mayadi. These were not somber conversations. The children joked and played with language in attempts to one-up each other in their harsh descriptions of compounds. When Samson said that the houses in the compounds had "grass on top," the children laughed loudly. Musa and Agnes added to the hilarity in their descriptions of "dirty" people and "even rats." The distinction implies the sizable differences between the environments in which the children live and those that they hear about from a distance. I interpreted their laughter and one-upmanship as a tactic to bond over the judgments in such terminology and implications of what such a reality meant in their own lives.

In its everyday usage in George, the compound-mayadi distinction is used to discipline and teach lessons to children. This became evident one afternoon as Olivious and I chatted with Angela and Julia in the tight passageway between their houses. Thirty-three-year-old Angela was born in George and her parents were longtime residents. She and her husband lived with their youngest daughter, eight-year-old Faustina, and Angela's sister's daughter, twelve-year-old Grace. Angela's ten-year-old son lived nearby with Angela's parents. Julia came from a neighboring country, settling in George where her sister also lived, marrying a local man, and becoming a mother to four children. She and Angela had struck up an enduring friendship.

Julia, Angela, Olivious, and I stood in the corridor, catching up on recent events while Faustina, Grace, and Julia's eight-year-old daughter, Aggie, sat underfoot on a reed mat, listening intently to our conversation. During a pause in gossip, I asked Angela: "So are the children [referring to Grace, Faustina, and Angela's son who lived with her parents] going on holiday this school break?" I was using the English word "holiday" in the way that I heard people in George use it to refer to the one- to two-week trips that children take to relatives' houses during their school breaks. Angela responded with laughter. She took a breath and said: "No, where are they supposed to go?" I silently thought about all of the places the children might go. They might go to Grace's mother's house in another residential area in Lusaka, or they could go to their grandmother's house in Kaunda Square, which they had visited on holiday before.

My thoughts were cut short as Angela continued: "All of us are in George." Julia broke in with a jokingly accusatory tone: "Why do you dislike George so much, *imwe* [you]? What? Do you want the kids to go to mayadi?" Angela countered: "I can't hate George. I'm from George. The kids are from George, and they will spend their lives in George." Unconvinced, Julia turned to Grace: "Do you want to see your mother [who lives] in mayadi?" Grace hesitated as they waited for her response. She shyly shook her head to indicate that she did not want to go to mayadi. The message in Julia's statement was expressed often in George. People who live in or desire to live in mayadi are viewed as proud, self-important people who think they are better than those around them. However, lessons learned and reinforced in such discussions are shifting and context dependent because many people also desire to get out of the compound. Adults used socio-spatial references also as a rhetorical device for disciplining children, persuading them to go to school, or teaching them particular lessons about manners. This aspect came out in the children's response to my question: children in mayadi throw nshima in the bin and not on the ground.

The children who described compounds in the workshop as places where people are illiterate and dirty and children behave poorly also actively worked against such impressions in defining their lives. They emphasized schooling, good behavior, and appearances. They demanded that I pay attention to the beauty and fun in their lives. In their drawings, the children showed themselves dressed up for Christmas and birthday parties, eating nice meals with families, taking family photos in newly purchased clothing, carrying out house chores with pride, and playing with friends and toys. They drew hearts, flowers, and symbols that stood for love. They wrote sentences in English, such as "I love this house" and "House is the best," next to drawings of their houses.

From an outside perspective, the homes they depicted looked decrepit. They had few windows and little room for the number of people residing in them. The floors were cracking and furniture was breaking down. In their drawings, the children did not point out the cracked floors or broken-down furniture. Instead, they highlighted the positive details of their homes.[10] The first drawing that ten-year-old Alick made for me showed rows of green plastic cups hung next to a family photo on a wall in his one-room home.[11] The cups came from his father's workplace where he manufactured plastic goods. Another boy, Mulenga, frequently mentioned and illustrated the red veranda that his mother polished daily (see fig. 1.3). Such small details in their drawings and daily lives showed that they were cared for; they were signs of the love that parents, grandparents, and other kin had for them.

Spatial terms, and the ways in which they are invoked by a range of local and global actors, teach children what is possible for them and valued. The meanings such terms take on can offer harsh judgments about behaviors and relationships. The terms exclude the things that make life beautiful and meaningful. Children's depiction of their environment both betrays and responds to simplistic descriptors such as compound or, in other parts of the world, slum, shantytown, squatter settlement, or blighted area. The children demonstrated how socio-spatial language can conflate poverty and a lack of resources with individual failure, poor behavior, and poor relationships. Such language can both fuel and dampen children's ambitions and dreams for the future and shape the ways in which children respond to their environment and their life's challenges.

DEVELOPMENT AND INEQUALITY ON THE GROUND

Since its development, residents of George have experienced both chronic shortages and development efforts to address such shortages. Public institutions continue to be overcrowded and under-resourced, and many services are unpredictable or only nominally provided. Lorries carrying *chibuku* (a low-alcohol beer distributed in giant plastic vats) are a more frequent presence than garbage trucks. The resource shortages and inequalities residents face become most visible during the rainy season when diseases flourish, roads become impassable, and mud is everywhere. Rubber boots provide some protection, but they are an unaffordable luxury for most residents and are worn mostly by men and then almost only when provided by their job. Most residents, including the very young, frail, and elderly, demonstrate enviable agility as they jump to and from rocks placed strategically across flooded areas. More than once, I slipped off of rocks or jumped too short and ended up splattering myself with mud. Onlookers observed my attempts at navigating flooded roads with amusement and offered

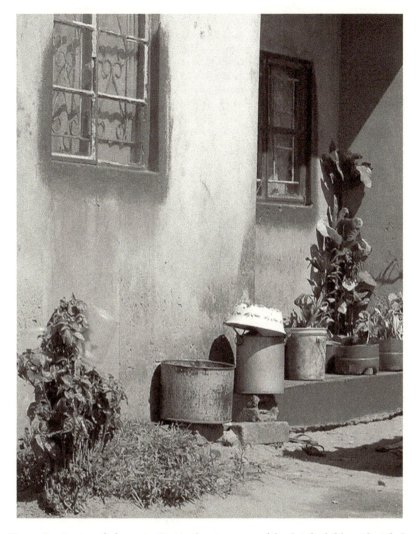

Fig. 1.3 Front entry of a house in George showing some of the details children identified with pride. The entryway and flowerpots were polished in a deep red. The windows were outlined with the same red polish. Photo by Rosha Forman.

lively commentaries on the perils of life in George, compared with life in other parts of the city, or in my home country.

Residents view Zambia's publicly operated electricity company, ZESCO, as reaffirming the large class disparities across Lusaka. George faces frequent and unpredictable power outages. In 2007 and 2008, these outages were lasting for days. Residents, including those without electrified homes, saw themselves as the clear losers in the distribution of power across the city.[12] Unpredictable outages

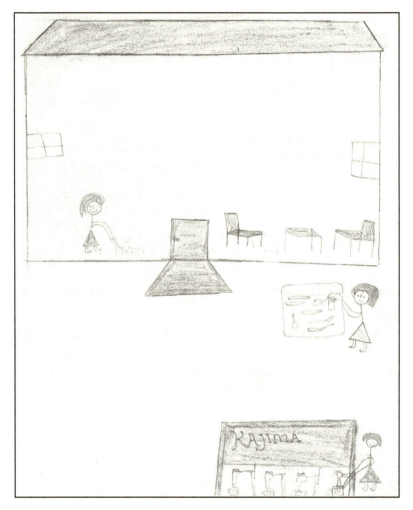

Fig. 1.4 Illustration of the household division of labor by age and gender. The mother goes to the kajima while the daughters stay home to sweep the house and wash dishes. Drawing by Irene, age twelve.

disrupted daily life. They cut people off from favorite television programs and news broadcasts, angering many who wanted to keep up-to-date on current affairs. Power outages at night shortened the time available to read, study, and socialize. Freezers defrosted in the absence of power, spoiling food in shops and homes, and contributing to lost money and income. When the government health center experienced extended outages, people either went without medical care or were forced to make expensive, time-consuming trips to private clinics or government-run clinics outside of George.

In a comical display one afternoon in 2008, there was even a power outage during a ZESCO-sponsored concert featuring a popular Zambian singer, JK. The concert was intended to promote responsible use of electricity, such as unplugging unused appliances. JK was a celebrity in Zambia and his music regularly blared from taverns and radios around the settlement. However, his live performances were out of reach for many residents who could not afford the expense. Without electricity, JK was unable to perform, disappointing the children and adults who gathered in anticipation of his concert.

When in 2008 a small group of residents staged a protest to draw attention to the lengthy power outages they were experiencing, a local television station covered the protest. The power company took notice. For at least a few months, power cuts in George were shorter and followed a much more predictable schedule than outages in the high-cost neighborhood where I lived. This short-lived win inspired hope for a better future. For some residents, it validated a belief that George would one day receive the amenities associated with higher- and middle-income residential areas, amenities such as a petrol station, bank, and supermarket.

The promise of change and the shortfall in efforts to develop George become especially evident in several areas—clean water, housing, schooling, and public health education—which are prioritized as part of development agendas and as part of poverty reduction strategies.

Clean Water

There have been some improvements in infrastructure in George since the 1990s, most notably in the water system, the largest development project in the settlement since upgrading in the 1970s. The *kajima* system—a system of protected standpipes distributed throughout George—was constructed in the 1990s with assistance from the Japanese development agency, JICA. The standpipes were constructed to reduce the high levels of cholera and other waterborne diseases in the settlement, which came from water in shallow wells and other unprotected sources. According to one report (JICA 2004), cholera was the cause of death for a staggering 70 in every 10,000 individuals in George in 1994. By 2000, mortality from cholera had fallen dramatically to 1 in every 10,000 individuals. A total of 386 kajimas, large communal cement structures with clean piped water, are in use across George. People talked about the kajimas as life-changing in ways that reminded me of my neighbor's lament when I served as a Peace Corps volunteer in rural Zambia. He said: "AIDS is better than cholera." In just one sentence, this young man showed how resource shortages exacerbate the incidence and suffering from multiple diseases, leading people to construct disease hierarchies.

The children admired the standpipes, and adults viewed them as a most outstanding example of international research and development in George. In their drawings, the children drew kajimas so often that it would take quite some effort to count the number of taps represented in their self-initiated drawings and in the margins of other assignments. I was surprised, then, when children did not incorporate kajimas into their maps of George. One boy drew a picture of himself with a bucket of water on his head. This water, he explained, that he had drawn from a shallow well. Another boy positioned himself at a communal standpipe in Matero, a neighboring residential area. This standpipe was not part of the recently constructed kajima system.

The absence of the kajimas in children's maps points to the reality that kajimas were not places for children, whose presence was, if not outright forbidden, strongly discouraged. I was told that, when the kajimas were constructed, the tap leaders, local residents who monitored water distribution, were instructed not to allow children to draw water. This practice derived from international concerns with child rights and exploitation as well as concerns that children would break the taps or make them dirty. Tap leaders varied in flexibility and, when Maureen became bedridden, she asked her tap leader to allow her twelve-year-old son, Kelvyn, to draw water. While Maureen was able to circumvent rules, most households were unable to work out such a flexible arrangement during crisis times.

The rules that forbade children from collecting water from kajimas were, in part, products of global discourses on child labor and child rights. While children in my study could not define the concept of child rights, most children offered that it was a child's right not to draw water. They did not offer this observation as an excuse to avoid water collection but as an observation; they had heard the term in conjunction with the concept of child rights. Children found other ways of procuring water for their households. Twelve-year-old Mary and her friends eagerly explained how they bypassed the system by hiding near the kajima and carrying water collected by an adult the rest of the way home. The adult would return to the kajima, collect another bucket, and the children would meet her again and so on. In these ways children resisted the global ideas about children's roles and responsibilities. Most of the time, and especially during dire and financially insecure times, children circumvented the system by drawing water from unregulated shallow wells, the very water points that the kajima system was meant to replace because they harbor disease. Sarafina did this and so did brothers Alick and Joe when their mothers were sick with TB and bedridden. Adding strain to households facing illness and other difficult circumstances, kajimas were fee paying. Women pointed out how stretched their household resources were and, in lean times, they could not afford the monthly fee. They, instead, paid smaller amounts to buy kajima water by the bucket and used water from shallow wells, even though they knew this water harbored diseases.

At the same time as the kajima system accomplished a change in local understandings of child rights and labor, it also reinforced that it was a woman's responsibility to provide water for their households, both through their labor and with their money (see fig. 1.4). When further asked about the difference between a woman and a girl, nine-year-old Kathryn responded: "Girls go to school; women go to draw water." Gift identified the difference as: "Women go to collect water but girls only sweep the outside."[13] The kajimas have created positive change in George, but my observations also demonstrate how well-intentioned policies can conflict with household needs, making the most vulnerable households and people even more vulnerable.

Housing

Housing is hugely overcrowded in George. An average household is composed of six people (three under age eighteen years) who share a living space of less than three rooms.[14] Housing types vary from single-room units, lined up in a row and purposely constructed to accommodate temporary residents, to larger houses with shaded porches. Even the smallest houses are often subdivided so that owners can rent out space. Such tight living conditions become most problematic at night when people have to share beds, sleep on couches, and set up temporary beds on floors in all rooms of the home. I knew several householders who sent children to sleep in houses of neighbors to relieve crowding.

Many houses in George do not have windows. They were either built without windows or the windows were filled in with mud bricks when owners could no longer afford glass windowpanes and burglar bars. Only a very few homes in a wealthier section of the residential area have inside running water. Most people draw water from the kajimas or from nearby shallow wells. A private pit latrine is a luxury, and most households in George share latrines among a number of neighbors.

Houses regularly flood in the rainy season. Water rushes through doors or seeps up from the oversaturated ground. Walls fall down. Toilets collapse. Flooding can happen at any time of the day, but its effects are most disastrous in the darkness of night, when people are least able to protect themselves and their things or gather neighbors to help. The mornings after a flood are tiring because of lost sleep and the hard labor of cleaning the house.

Children play primary roles in returning flooded houses to their previous condition. For example, I arrived at the Simwondes' house one morning to find ten-year-old Mulenga mucking out mud and water that filled their sitting room. He had gathered his close-knit group of friends to help. On a different day, I arrived at the Katongos' house in time to observe the exhaustion caused by the rains. The entire household sat outside in weary silence. Too tired to do anything else, Joe Katongo and his brother Alick skipped school and their father stayed home from work.

Land to build new houses has run short in George. Residents and newcomers fill in the gaps. They add on to their houses and build structures between existing homes, and they construct new housing at the margins of the settlement. The land at the border was once low-lying, flood-prone bush. Now it is filled with houses. On one side of the settlement, new housing and burial plots have literally converged.

The meeting of home and resting place unsettled mourners, including myself when I attended the burial of Patrick Njovu in 2007. Walking from road to burial site, we stepped over plots marked off for housing construction. These new houses sat just meters from dozens of burial plots that were dug that week. Mourners gossiped about corrupt government officials who sold uninhabitable housing plots to make quick money. They questioned the legality of the housing and whether the people who bought them would own the plots. And we all doubted that anyone would want to build there. Months later, I attended another burial. This time, the burial ground was scheduled to be closed down to new burials, and residents wondered where they would bury their dead. Problems of land for the urban poor do not disappear when they die.

Because of land shortages and also because of the expenses associated with building a house, home ownership is not available to everyone in George. In my survey of 200 households, 75 respondents owned their houses, 105 rented houses, and 20 stayed for free in a house owned by someone who lived elsewhere. Homeowners lived in George for more than twice as long as renters, and their owning came with marked advantages. Ownership frees people from the whims and rules of landlords, who may leave property in disrepair, raise rents unexpectedly, or evict renters without reason. Home ownership enables owners to, instead, become landlords, and many homeowners in George divide and rent out sections of their houses for income. Ownership also has other social and economic benefits. Owners are able to host visitors and funerals. They are able to sell fruits, vegetables, charcoal, cigarettes, beer, and frozen treats from their homes, activities which landlords often forbid. And because wage labor opportunities in Zambia are biased toward men, these economic activities most frequently benefited women and children, as I will describe in more detail in chapter 2.

Women face particular challenges in attaining housing security in George, particularly when they live in houses owned by their husbands. Husbands tend to hold on to property and expect a woman's maternal relatives to provide for her in cases of divorce. When I first met Julia, she told me about this "trouble with men." Even though her marriage appeared stable, she said that she could never know exactly what her husband was doing. Months later her husband moved out of the house to live with his girlfriend. He made his move on the day Julia went to the clinic to give birth to their fourth child. When Julia returned from the clinic with her new baby on her back, she learned that her husband wanted her out of the house. His brothers, who shared ownership of the house because the house had belonged to their parents, convinced him to let her stay, though this was a temporary reprieve. Soon Julia's husband moved her into a small unit of another house owned by his family. The last time I met Julia, we sat on the floor of this unfurnished house. She told me that he had threatened to throw her out of that house too, and he was not contributing anything to the care of her children. Yet she was unsure that any good would come from taking him to the Victim Support Unit at the local police station.[15]

The insecurities women face when their husbands die are similarly acute. Customary inheritance practices in Zambia give a man's maternal relatives ownership of the property they leave behind. This can leave his wife and children with few claims to a house and other assets and with no place to go. In 1989, Zambia passed the Intestate Succession Act to address, legally, the vulnerability of women and children to such property grabbing by a deceased husband's family. The law grants women and children rights to houses when a husband or father dies. Still, in George and elsewhere in Zambia, lingering ideologies about men's ownership of property have rendered this act largely ineffective (Hansen 1997). In the courts used by residents of George, the law was only first applied fifteen years after it passed (Schlyter 2009), and I knew a number of women who were left homeless, "without even a bed" as one woman phrased it, when their husbands died. As Julia's experience suggests, women continue to have little success in retaining property, even with the support of the court system.

When women get ownership of houses in urban Zambia, they typically hold on to their houses (Hansen 1997). In my sample of 200 households in George, women made up only 23 percent of the household heads. However, female heads of household accounted for nearly 50 percent of the home owners in my survey.

Home ownership is not always what it may seem, and there are substantial constraints that come with ownership for women, in particular. Many houses in George are shared among family members after the owner dies and leaves the house to several of their grown children. In such cases, widowed or divorced women and their children may keep up houses while brothers or more well-off and married sisters live elsewhere. This may give them more security and greater chances to generate income. However, they are also subject to the demands of relatives. They must host frequent visitors, make repairs, and maintain the house. As one woman told me, the crux of her problem was that she did not have a house to pass down to her children when she died because she did not singularly own it. In contrast, her brothers were building homes of their own for their children. This, she pointed out, created further differences between the life chances of her children in George and the children her brothers were raising in more affluent neighborhoods in Lusaka.

Schooling

Both boys and girls focused heavily on schools in their map drawings. This was, in part, because schools were everywhere in the settlement. Just as residents used the kajima water system to point out development in George, they also noted the recent influx of schools as a positive change. On my first visit to George in 2005, I, too, was struck by how many schools there were: seven government schools, forty-four private schools, and around forty community schools. It seemed that, with so many schools, this was one area where there was no shortage of national and international attention.

The high number of schools was an outcome of global efforts to make universal basic education available to children in even the poorest and remotest areas of the world. In 2002, the Zambian Ministry of Education declared that government basic school would be offered at no fee to students, citing cost as a reason for low enrollment and rising dropout rates (Ministry of Education 2010). By 2005, basic education enrollment in Zambia had grown from 1.7 million to 2.8 million children. While the numbers suggest great success, the influx of children surpassed educational resources, placing a sizable strain on schools and significant overcrowding in classrooms.

It was an incredible achievement to enroll a child in the government basic schools in George. Around 26 percent of George's population was between the ages of six and fourteen in 2008, and there were only seven government schools. Residents talked about the lengths they went to enroll their children in these schools. They waited in long queues to attain spots for children. They sent children to live with grandparents or other relatives who lived closer to a government school or had the social connections needed to secure the child a spot. Efforts to get children into government schools at times rested on subterfuge. Julia, for example, bought her eight-year-old daughter a placement in a government school from another child's parents. The first time I drew with Julia's daughter, the girl made me drawings of flowers and houses. When her daughter paused to think about what to draw next, Julia suggested, "Write your school name for Ba Jeannie." She wrote her school name—the other young girl's name—with ease and confidence. When I asked her to write her own name, she struggled to spell it.

Because of the inaccessibility and insufficiency of government basic schools, nongovernmental and private education providers play an increasingly large role in providing schooling in George. Whereas private schools provide education at varying costs, community schools are intended to cater to the most vulnerable children, especially girls and children affected by HIV and AIDS. However, community schools are not always free of costs. Some ask for contributions that resemble school fees, blurring the line between community and private schooling for many residents.

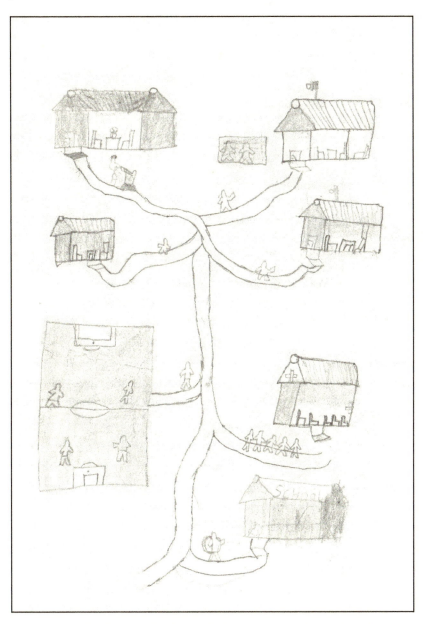

Fig. 1.5 Map of all of the places Stephen regularly goes. His map shows a football field, his church, and the houses of friends and relatives. Stephen drew himself at the bottom going to school. Drawing by Stephen, age eleven.

The push for children to attend primary school and the availability of different schooling options has meant that many children in George are enrolled in school. However, enrollment does not indicate the quality of education or whether or not a child attends school. Almost every school in George has interruptions and days missed due to factors such as water and power shortages, the illness or death of a teacher, the social obligations teachers face to attend funerals of fellow teachers, and much more. Additionally, many children in private and fee-paying community schools are "chased" away from school, temporarily suspended for nonpayment of school fees, at the beginning and middle of each term. They are not allowed back until they pay their school fees. Even children in government schools, who do not have to pay school fees, are chased when they do not have a proper uniform and shoes or basic school supplies, such as a pencil and notebooks.

The children's emphasis on schools in their drawings was partially because going to school was an aspect of daily life, and partially due to the struggles children faced in accessing a good education (see fig. 1.5). The children who had the most insecurity in their schooling tended to place greater emphasis on schools in their drawings. Even children who did not attend school drew schools in prominent places on their maps of George. In their map drawings, the two children who were out of school the longest situated themselves on the outside of schools, looking in.

Accessing a good education has become part of children's everyday struggles to make a good life for themselves. In a tape-recorded exercise in which children told stories based on pictures I provided, ten-year-old Abby Banda offered an account of the predicament that she and many children face in George.[16] Looking at a drawing of a boy who was carrying a bag and wearing short pants, a tailored shirt, and (as most children pointed out) very nice shoes, Abby spoke into my tape recorder:

> Here I see this boy going to school. If he finishes school, goes to college, does everything well, he starts a well-paid job to feed his family and provides everything because you will have money. You can even get a house for the family— that is, your wife and children, so that you also send them to school so that they also get educated but also to take care of him when he is aged. [Long pause.] This boy wants to be educated just like a lot of pupils. But insufficient funds. There is a problem. Even me, I want school, but it is because of the same problem. I do not know when I will start again or even if I will ever finish school or not. That's what, what I have seen on this picture.

Abby borrowed from international and national advocacy discourses that placed a premium on education as the key to economic security and future success. In other recordings, Abby talked about the importance of education for girls.

Abby linked education to housing and viewed a good education as a means for her to control her future. With an education, Abby observed, a woman can buy a house and avoid the insecurities women face in marriage. She said, "Instead, you chase him [your husband from your home]. Not him chasing you [from his home] in the middle of the night." Abby later told me: "If you hate school, life will also hate you." She believed that a good education was not just for her own individual benefit, but also the way for her to fulfill her obligations to her mother, younger siblings, and her own future children.

It was a cruel irony that, several months later, Abby found herself living in a school, but only briefly attending it. Her mother's brother, with whom she was living, rented their house to a man interested in starting a private school. They painted the wall around the house in bright colors and put up extra pit latrines for the children. Abby's uncle moved out, leaving Abby with her mom and two younger siblings. Abby started attending the school, but quickly stopped. The family remained silent concerning why Abby stopped attending the school after only several days, saying that they wanted her to transfer to a government school.

Transferring between the different types of schools constituted a way of hedging one's bets by keeping children in schools of varying costs, distances, and qualities for specific lengths of time rather than taking them out of school completely. By age fourteen, 68 percent of children I surveyed across 200 households had changed schools at least once. The main reasons for transferring were expense (33 percent), quality of the education (21 percent), distance due to a move (19 percent), and distance when there was no move (10 percent). My ethnographic observations in Abby's and other children's households affirm that these answers were accurate, and they also demonstrated that the expense and moves related to illness and death were primary motivators for school transfers.

The practice of transferring among schools was so common that Alick included the following in a story he based on the same picture to which Abby referred when she described the importance of school for future success. Alick said: "Here I'm going to Muchinga [Government Basic] School myself. I met a friend [in the road]. I asked him which school are you at now? He told me he's at Lilanda [Government Basic] School. Then I wondered how many times is he going to change [schools]." Alick hinted in his story that transferring among schools too frequently could indicate larger problems in the family. Children and adults almost always discussed children's time out of school as a temporary, rather than permanent, situation. They referred to it in terms of transferring to a less expensive, higher quality, or closer school or waiting on a relative to provide money. In an environment where schooling is now considered to be accessible and free, I found that guardians unable to provide schooling for their children blamed themselves, and children experienced stigma associated with school leaving.

Within the push for universal basic education, a strong national and international discourse has positioned schooling as a child's right and a moral issue. It suggested to children like Abby that schooling was their route out of poverty. My observations point to the difficulties families faced and the lengths they went so that their children enroll and remain in school. The starkest examples of these efforts was transferring among schools and, as we saw earlier, buying other children's government school placements.

Many factors aside from enrollment prevented children from actually receiving the education that they worked so hard to achieve. Despite their efforts, most children in my study were not able to read or write very well, if at all. This was indicative of larger trends in the country, in which more children were enrolled in and completing school, but literacy rates were falling (Kelly 2008).[17] This disconnect between school enrollment and literacy rates demands attention to the quality of schooling children receive as well as the factors driving contemporary transfer rates, rather than simply counting enrollment as a success. The influx of private and nongovernmental schools into George has been a welcome change to no schooling. However, my evidence suggests that families were tactically school hopping among these institutions in the hopes of securing an education for their children. As it stands now, the promise of schooling as the answer to poverty is a false one for many children in George.

Public Health Education

When I was a Peace Corps volunteer in Lundazi, Zambia, I lived near a school from 1999 to 2001 that had the motto "No sweet without sweat." The motto seemed particularly apt in a place where sweets were in fact in very short supply. Of course, the intended meaning of the motto was that hard work and struggle are necessary to attain the good things in life. As I think of the mottos I saw on schools after this time, I am reminded of how HIV and AIDS and also the discourses that surround disease prevention have become such an integral part of children's daily lives (see fig. 1.6). HIV messages were everywhere in George, broadcast as part of school mottos and also on children's bodies when schools used HIV messaging as part of their uniforms.

HIV has affected all aspects of formal educational, from a child's ability to actually attend school to the quality of teaching and the content of lesson plans (Cliggett and Wyssmann 2009). The presence of HIV has also shaped the urgency with which health-related messages and lessons are incorporated in and on schools. The lessons children received in and on schools were meant for the children, and they were also intended for adults living in the children's households and community. Through school-based programs, children were asked to distribute public health messages in many ways.[18] The success of such programs has rested on children's abilities to repeat correct biomedical information and their willingness to distribute such knowledge.

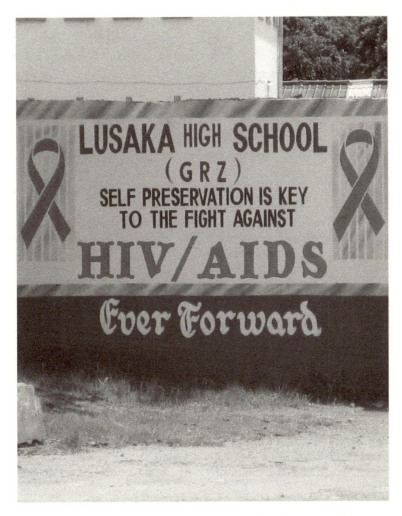

Fig. 1.6 School sign with HIV messaging, 2008. Photo by Eric Donohue.

HIV messaging was also used as a tool to fund schools in George. Many children in the households I worked with were required to purchase specific t-shirts to wear on Fridays. Take for example the private school that Regina attended. Her school's t-shirt said the name of the school and "Fight HIV/AIDS." It cost around US$9. Because Regina's aunt could not afford to buy the t-shirt for Regina or her own daughter and son, the children were chased from school each Friday for not wearing the appropriate attire. The children eventually took to skipping school on Fridays, in the absence of an alternative.

Given the focus on HIV-related issues that affect young people in Zambia and the explicit governmental push to incorporate HIV education into school curricula, I was surprised when children in my study said that they did not learn about HIV or TB in school. Even after much probing and some very leading questions, the children still did not discuss school programs concerning TB education. Few mentioned learning about HIV in schools.[19]

When asked where they learned about HIV and TB, the children listed "the road." Children reported learning about TB from a vehicle that drove around George and effortlessly repeated the messages shouted over the megaphone from the truck: "Go to George clinic and get tested. Men and women." They recounted NGO-sponsored drama performances on TB and HIV that they had seen in public spaces in the community. Such performances were not intended for children, but children were their main consumers (Bond et al. 2010). Recalling the children's map drawings, these findings are not unsurprising. The children denoted in their drawings roads of varying sizes and shapes, with distance marked by curvy lines. These roads were dynamic places where the children met friends, gossiped, carried out chores, and sought diversions. In narrating their maps, I noticed that most children were less interested in telling me about places (homes, schools, and markets) than they were in describing roads and pathways, locating themselves and their friends in paths, and discussing what goes on in them. Their emphasis on roads bore similarities to Barry Percy-Smith's (2002) observations that British children create their own city spaces in undesignated areas, beyond parks, playgrounds, schools, and their homes. In this sense, the children in George were also creating their own spaces to learn about health and disease.

Much HIV and TB education, as well as education on a range of health behaviors, has focused in schools and on didactic lessons. A view of learning as only school-based misses out on important ways in which children acquire as well as distribute knowledge and come to understand disease prevention. As I will demonstrate in chapters 2 and 3, it also underestimates the broader constraints children face that may make such education ineffective and shape the ways in which children understand disease messaging, within the contexts of their lives.

Conclusion

This chapter has offered an important foundation for the following chapters, and it also bears relevance beyond an understanding of children's lives in one part of Zambia. There are broader lessons in a detailed analysis of the institutional and environmental context in which children live and participate. First, in George, as in poor urban settings around the world, children experienced a range of internationally driven projects designed with particular assumptions about childhood and children's needs. The assumptions embedded in such programming affect children's everyday lives in complicated, shifting, and also contested ways. The kajima standpipe example demonstrated one way in which children were finding new constraints and opportunities for action within international development projects. The kajima system significantly reduced the incidence of waterborne disease in George. There is little doubt that this contributed positively to children's well-being. The kajimas were well built, and the children were proud of them. Yet the same children were also excluded from using them by a policy that viewed children's collection of water as labor unfit for children and worried that children might dirty or ruin the water sources. The children were not passive and, when the rules did not fit their needs and the needs of their households, some children found ways to utilize the kajimas. However, not all children negotiated access to the kajimas and remained dependent upon shallow wells that were known to harbor diseases. This aspect stands as a warning that well-intended policies might not only be unproductive but also dangerous to children and their households. Their range of actions and pride around the kajimas show that the ethics of children's labor are complicated and contextual. They also demonstrate that children can be excluded from and also included in international projects at the same time.

In George, as I have shown, schools are overcrowded. There is only one government health center, and it, too, is overcrowded and under-resourced. Environmental conditions produce illness and uncertainty. Housing is difficult to secure and easily damaged; and amenities, such as electricity and trash collection, are provided with irregularity. The children lived with these shortages, as they lived with the stigma of growing up in the compound. The second lesson is on the lengths to which people go to maintain hope, secure resources, and make life livable under extreme constraint. The example of transferring schools showed one way in which residents attempted to do so. School enrollment is a development objective promoted by national and international actors and written into the United Nations Millennium Development Goals (MDGs), which identifies universal primary schooling as part of a larger blueprint for ending poverty. School enrollment may be easier in George than it was in the past because of the array of private and community schools and the removal of fees for government basic school. However, receiving a good education was a challenge. In a setting where family crises were frequent and schools varied in quality and expense, transferring schools became a tactic that many families used to attain schooling for their children. The ideology of schooling as the way out of poverty was strong, which Abby vividly showed. Transferring schools became a key way in which residents actively attempted to maintain hope and also manage uncertain futures.

The third lesson I learned from attentiveness to children may be the most unexpected for an outside observer. Many children noted the beauty in George, drawing trees, flowers, freshly polished floors, and tidy homes. How might we take into consideration objects of pride and beauty when addressing children's lives in a place like George? First, recognizing beauty and pride does not mean ignoring the problems. However, it does mean that we need to take more care with our language and characterizations so that we do not turn complex lives into caricatures. The children actively resisted the stereotypes about them that were signified by the term *compound*. They did so in the ways they focused on their schooling and proper behavior and also when they identified the positive aspects of their environments. Second, shifting the focus to what children find meaningful offers insight into how children also attempt to address their conditions, even if they are not successful in doing so. It honors their relationships and their attempts to maintain dignity within difficult circumstances. Finally, knowing the small signs that children look for and value forces us to recognize when these signs are absent. The children showed that an absence of small signs offered reason to be concerned about a child's well-being. As the children pointed out, an unpolished floor or untidy home, just as excessive transferring among schools, suggested a larger crisis in their households as well as a larger crisis within their families and relationships, which I now turn to in chapter 2.

CHAPTER 2

Residence and Relationships

I caught up to Maureen Nkhoma on the dirt road that ran in front of her house. During my initial visits with Maureen, she was so debilitated that she could barely stand on her own. Five months later, she was well enough to go to the *kajima* several times a day to draw water. She balanced a yellow jerry can filled with water on her head. Her neck muscles tensed as the container swayed when she stopped to greet me. Slapping my hand and holding it in hers, we greeted each other:

MAUREEN: *Mwauka bwanji, Jeanie?* [How did you wake?]
JEAN: *Bwino. Mwauka banji, Amake Loveness?* [I woke well. How did you wake, mother of Loveness?]

I asked how each of her children awoke that morning and how her mother, who was visiting from the family's farm, awoke. Everyone "woke well," except for her mother, whose legs were aching after the long bus ride to George. Maureen's eyes lit up as we turned to questions about my household:

MAUREEN: *Bauka bwanji ku nyumba?* [How did everyone awake at your house?]
JEAN: *Bauka bwino.* [They woke well.]
MAUREEN: *Bauka bwanji mpando?* [How did your chairs wake?]
JEAN: *Bauka bwino.* [They woke well.]
MAUREEN: *Na tebulo?* [And your table?]

This was an old joke between us, and we laughed every time. Maureen's jokes about my furniture started months before when she realized that I lived alone. My household set-up surprised her, and she advised me to keep [*kusunga*] a child. Maureen explained it this way: I spent long days in George and so I needed someone to clean the house, do my laundry, and make my meals. A child could help me with this work and forestall the loneliness that she knew I felt during the evenings and on Sundays, when I was not in George. Her references to my chairs, table, and material wealth were pointed. They identified the absence of people in my home and indexed my financial capacity to keep a child.

On this particular day, Maureen jokingly suggested that I keep Loveness, her eight-year-old daughter. Loveness, she said, listened well to adults, and she knew how to cook, clean the house, and wash dishes and clothes. Proof of her capabilities was in Maureen's house, which Loveness had kept clean during the worst of Maureen's illness. She talked about the things I needed to consider when keeping Loveness. Maureen said that I would, of course, find a school for Loveness near where I lived, and I would pay for all of Loveness's other needs. Maureen's jesting taught me two key facts of life: the resources and opportunities children are afforded depend on relationships, and children make day-to-day life meaningful and possible through their affective and practical actions. That is, interdependence characterized relations between adults and children.

I played along and emphasized that Loveness would refuse me (*akana maningi!*), to which Maureen laughed and replied that Loveness could not refuse the move; she was fond of me, and I had become family over the past few months of visiting them. By framing me as family, Maureen was giving me a lesson on moral expectations that family members help one another.[1] She subtly criticized my isolation and stinginess. She more openly criticized her own family members, claiming that Loveness had not received a thing from her relatives, not even an invitation to visit their house. It was unlikely that Maureen would have let Loveness move, even if family members had offered. She proved this point when her brother wanted her son to move in with him during a time when Maureen was still very ill. She asked: "Am I not his mother? He should stay with his mother." She followed this up by telling me how much her son provided her with care, something that she had also emphasized when we first met, as I described in the introduction.

At the time I write this book, observers of the HIV epidemic in sub-Saharan Africa, including policy makers, development practitioners, researchers, and the media, have expressed grave concerns about the capacities of families to care for children. It is often repeated that HIV has caused a crisis of care, in which there are not enough adult family members capable of providing care to children as there had been in the past. Such strains are deeply felt by people in George, as Maureen suggested when she criticized family members for not inviting Loveness to their house and, conversely, when she expressed resentment when family members invited her son to stay with them.

In this chapter, I examine this crisis of care by viewing children as actors in family networks. This approach offers a different analytic for understanding the crisis of care than is typically used in research and reports to assess children's needs. For example, typically, children's needs have been examined in terms of discrete outcomes, such as nutrition, school enrollment, and unpaid labor. These measures and others are correlated with whether children's biological parents are living or dead (often referred to as orphan status), the types of households in which children reside (grandparent-headed, woman-headed, child-headed), and if children are living outside of family care, in institutions or on the streets. Such measures acknowledge the importance of family care, but they cannot capture the dynamism of relationships, the mobility of children's lives, and the roles children play in families. My overarching goal in this chapter is to fill in gaps in our understandings of and approaches to family care, both of which drive humanitarian initiatives and policy prescriptions aimed at children. To achieve this goal, I examine how children and their adult family members thought about children's kin relationships and their roles in families. I pay careful attention to children's attempts to achieve good care for themselves within exceptionally difficult circumstances and within newer global discourses of childhood.

Economic Life in George

Material scarcity in George was a fact of life that structured the children's roles and relationships in and across households as well as their access to resources. Unemployment in formal sector work has continued to be high in Lusaka, especially in the low-cost settlements where many of Lusaka's poorest residents live. Only a fortunate few adults in my study—mostly men—found formal sector jobs in areas such as meat and dairy packing, road construction, and contract carpentry. These jobs were low paying with long hours. One of the highest earners made about US$80 a month as a security guard in Lusaka's industrial area, several kilometers outside of George. He worked every day of the week, with two days off per month. His job provided more security than most, though ultimately, his sickness undermined even this security. He was fired when his absences ran over his company's allotted sick leave.

While men struggled to find and keep formal sector work, women in George faced even greater challenges in the labor market because of their lower literacy rates than men, the preferential treatment men received from employers, and social expectations that women would remain close to home as caregivers and housewives (Schlyter 2009). Only one woman in my study worked a formal sector job. She attained her job through a male relative who knew the employer and advocated on her behalf. Most women made their living through cobbling together piecework and other informal labor activities, such as petty trading. They broke stones, worked with NGOs on the improvement projects that entered into the settlement, and sold food, goods, or services (such as hair plaiting or tailoring). Their work was time consuming and could be exhausting. One woman I knew woke at three o'clock every morning to walk several kilometers to a rural area where she bought vegetables to sell in George. She sat at her market stand during the day, remaining there until she sold the last of her vegetables at dusk. Another woman spent her days in Lusaka's town center carrying a basket of bananas on her head to sell to hungry passersby. Many women bought or made things to sell from their houses, such as fritters, grilled meats, frozen drinking water, and "ice block" (flavored ice in a bag).

The ways in which children participated in economic life were indicative of both the difficulties involved in making a living and the gendered inequalities in the labor market. In several group discussions, I asked the children to tell me their roles in economic life, using the question: "Do children provide food for the house?" In George, the phrase "providing food for the house" referred generally to a two-part process in which a person had money or other resources and shared these resources with other members of the household.[2] This question took into account that households, as feminist anthropologists have shown, can be sites of competition and differentiation, in which members compete over and negotiate access to resources, rights, and obligations (Moore 1994). Husbands and wives in Lusaka have not necessarily shared their earnings, with women frequently not knowing how much their husbands made (Hansen 1997). Further, women and their kin have borne primary responsibility for feeding and clothing children and ensuring that they attended school in ways that fathers and fathers' kin have not. Conceptualizing households as homogenous and discrete units when they are in actual fact differentiated and dynamic can conceal the complexity of relations among household members as well as among members of different households. Just as cultural and economic processes frame relations between men and women, they also frame relations between adults and children, particularly women and children.

My question to the children about whether and how they provided food for the household was aimed at understanding not just their contributions but how they envisioned themselves economically and within gendered and generational relations in the households:

JEAN: Do children provide food for the house?
GIFT: *Awe!* [No!] They just sit.
KATHRYN: Awe! They just sit.
FAUSTINA: Awe! They just eat.
MULENGA: Some play.
IRENE: Children go to school.

The children did sit at home, eat, play, and go to school, but they also did much more. Take Gift for example, the eight-year-old boy who first claimed, "*Awe!*

They just sit," in answer to my question. Gift carried out labor that, in my assessment, helped support two households in his family. Despite Gift's small size, he was very "strong," a term his grandmother invoked frequently in reference to his capabilities. Gift accompanied his grandmother to the family's farm for weeks at a time to help with planting and harvesting. When he was in George, he did many other things: swept, washed dishes, went to the market to buy food for his mother and grandmother, and ran errands for his uncle, who repaired cars. He drew water from a shallow well in his parents' yard to sell to neighbors, who paid him by the bucket. He followed his bus driver father to the bus queuing area, where he sat on a low-lying wall, conveying messages, doling out information, and directing bus traffic for his father.

Given the amount of work that Gift and other children accomplished, how do we interpret phrases such as sitting, eating, and playing? Analyses of similar statements made by youth in Lusaka and farther afield in Accra, Ghana, offer some clues. In Karen Tranberg Hansen's (2005) research with youth in Lusaka, she has called such phrases "discursive metaphors." Metaphors such as "sitting at home," she argued, offer insight into how the youth felt about being stuck in the compounds without opportunities for spatial or socioeconomic mobility. Drawing on Hansen's work, Thilde Langevang and Katherine Gough (2009) have shown how young people in Ghana used such phrasing to characterize their positions within a labor market that had largely shut them out. Their primary focus was to "not spend too much time 'sitting at home' and 'eating' as this signals unemployment, laziness and consumption rather than accumulation" (749). Daily movement around the city became a key strategy for survival and attempt to cultivate personal success through seeking out work and creating social networks.

The children in my study referred to eating, sitting, and playing from their own particular social positions, which differed from those of the youth in Hansen's and Langevang and Gough's studies. Most of the work that children accomplished both supported women in their activities and was directed by women. In my survey of children's activities in households in George, the majority of the 313 children ages six to fourteen carried out domestic chores in households and other activities that helped women most directly with their social expectations and labor market work. Most of the 313 children watched younger children in the household, washed dishes, and swept the house regularly. A quarter of the children assisted with market-based activities in their households, through their help selling goods out of their houses or watching an *ntemba* [small shop or stand] set up next to the house. Fewer children—only 28 out of 313—were reported as regularly helping with market activities away from the house, in the markets or "the field" (walking around the settlement selling food that they carried in a basket).

Children also supported women during a household illness through all of the above activities as well as through the nursing care they provided. Of the 313 children counted by the survey, 262 were said to collect medicine to give to the sick members of their households. However, while the children acknowledged that they did these activities, they did not necessarily consider them as their own work. Let me illustrate this point through ten-year-old Chipo's response to a question I asked in one of the children's workshops. I asked the children a question about who in a house takes care of a sick person. My intention was to disentangle children's ideas about their roles in caregiving activities. Ten-year-old Chipo, who lived in one of the comparison households (without a TB patient at the time of the study), proudly announced: "Mary's mother takes care of the sick." Chipo lived in a large household with her mother, father, and a number of older siblings and their children. Mary was Chipo's niece, who was two years older than Chipo. When I asked Chipo what Mary's mother did to give care, Chipo gave this hypothetical response: "She makes Mary help the sick by giving him the medicine, washing clothes, cleaning in the home and washing plates in the home and sweeping the home."

Children supported their households through domestic work, helped with income-generating endeavors, and cared for the sick, but their opportunities to accumulate resources for themselves or their households were limited. Only 16 out of 313 children in my survey were reported to carry out piecework, such as crushing stones or other odd jobs, on a consistent basis. This low number was due in part to the actual availability of work in George; competition for even the lowest-paying piecework was great. There was also significant shame in George associated with children's performance of labor, which many children and adults perceived as inappropriate for young children to perform year round or for the household's benefit, though they made exceptions when such work occurred between school terms and was aimed at raising money for school expenses.

Children relied on adults to meet their basic needs, and this dependence came with expectations that they would contribute to household labor. Such expectations included sitting at home in order to respond to the fluctuating needs of the household, which varied by household composition, season, and other events and crises, such as sickness or the birth of a new baby.[3] This practice became even more evident during the illness of a household member. Rose, for example, made a drawing of her grandmother lying outside on a reed mat, with Rose sitting by her side looking at her. Monica told me that she gave her mother everything she wanted so that she could get better. Mary, as Chipo observed, responded to her mother's orders to care for the sick. By remaining close, children were best positioned to observe and then react to household needs as they arose.

The children most often expressed pride in their help around the house, but they at times actively resisted such work or the demands that they stay at home in case there was work for them to carry out. They resisted by leaving their houses to avoid both hearing and needing to respond to adults' requests. Still, the children knew that leaving for long periods of time each day without a reason, such as going to school or running an errand, carried risks. Such absences could lead to discord between them and other members of their household, particularly women, if the child's help was needed and the children were nowhere to be seen. Recall my conversation with the children about whether they provide food for the household. Mulenga said that "some [children] play." The tone of his statement carried moral evaluation, with playing too much viewed as naughty.

Whereas Langevang and Gough (2009) found that sitting at home implied laziness and consumption for the youth in their study, the opposite was true for younger children in George. The children I knew suggested that moving around too much during the day could be a sign of laziness and consumption.[4] The children described that some children played away from the house a lot and only returned home when they wanted to eat, which they saw as both disobedient and risky. It was risky because adults did not always share their food with children, particularly when they were annoyed with them. This annoyance frequently extended, at least in the children's viewpoints, from an adult's impression that the child was either naughty or lazy or that they consumed too many resources already. So as not to give such an impression, children limited their daily mobility and remained close to home, at least when adults were present. During illness, sitting at home—and staying close to particular relatives—acquired further significance as it enabled children to accommodate a range of needs of the ill person and of any women who might be caring for that person.

Anthropologist Tobias Hecht's (1998) work offers insight for interpreting children's domestic efforts. In a study of street children in Brazil, he contrasted two types of what he referred to as "home children" (as opposed to "street children"): children who were nurtured and children who nurtured. He suggested that, in Brazil, the children of the rich experienced nurtured childhood, while children of the poor experienced childhood through the acts they engaged in to nurture and bring resources into their households. Hecht identified this as a central difference between rich and poor childhoods in Brazil: "Whereas nurtured children are loved by virtue of *being* children, the love received by nurturing children is to a great extent a function of what they *do*" (1998, 80). In George, childhood might be considered through this framework, with children most frequently fitting Hecht's nurturing childhood description. Yet the children in my study were not wholly independent, as Hecht has suggested of nurturing children in Brazil. The children not only expected to do things for adults, but they derived value and benefits from doing them, including the affective and material inputs of adults. These may not be actions particular to childhood, but to vulnerability and marginalization in the labor market in general.[5]

My description of children's household activities suggests that we cannot conceptualize children in George as either dependent or independent. Adults, too, could not be considered independent, especially when they relied so heavily upon children's support to make their livings and maintain households. I find it much more accurate to characterize the relationship between the children and adults as one of interdependence (Bray and Brandt 2007). This interdependence, as both Maureen's jest and Gift's activities have shown, was not limited to people living within a singular household but also occurred across households. Just because children and adults relied upon one another did not mean that they had equal or reciprocal relationships. People in George—both young and old— thought deeply about their interdependencies as well as the inequalities in their relationships, particularly when deciding where children were kept and what constituted good care for children versus exploitation or suffering. This became particularly evident in decisions and debates about children's movements among the households in their extended family.

Keeping Children Is Hard, Necessary, and Helpful

The HIV epidemic has caused much speculation on changes to family unity and generosity due to the economic and caregiving strains that morbidity and premature deaths place on families. Early scholars of African kinship systems identified kin solidarity as a moral ideal that underpinned the relations of consanguines, kin related to one another through common blood.[6] Anthropologist Elizabeth Colson reinforced this view with her observation that in Zambia during times of hunger, people "walk many miles to beg from kinsmen living in villages where there is some hope of finding food. These [kinsmen] may grumble, but so long as anything remains in their granaries or they have funds with which to purchase grain, they are likely to divide with their indigent relatives" (1958, 21). Kin generosity extended to the social parenting of children, and children circulated frequently among kin to spread out the costs of child rearing, receive schooling, provide work in households, and receive instruction from many relatives, and not just their biological parents.[7]

A longstanding body of research on children's circulation in Zambia and elsewhere in sub-Saharan Africa has identified that children belonged to many households. To quote Colson once more: "The majority of children by the time they have reached puberty have had the experience of adjusting themselves to life in a strange household, and a portion of their training has been received from outside the immediate family" (1958, 258). This does not mean that kin were always generous with children or that kin never exploited children's efforts, as Hansen (1990) has shown in archival research on children's labor in urban Zambia during the colonial and postcolonial eras. Rather, the ideal of kin generosity in sharing children across households and providing for the children of kin was a principle through which people assessed the strength of their relationships, their own virtue, and the virtue of their kin.

Researchers and practitioners have questioned the effects of HIV on people's abilities to keep and care for children in the African countries most affected by HIV, and have revised their understandings of children's circulation in the context of HIV. Some researchers have identified children's circulation as a critical household and family coping strategy within the epidemic.[8] Others have observed that children have fewer sources of support and places to go because of the caregiving and economic strains HIV places on households.[9] In my observations, such processes were co-occurring, rather than competing, as children were staying in place and moving, and they provided relief to households in crisis while also burdening them. Take the following case of the Simwondes as an example.

Vailless Simwonde rubbed her hands down her legs as she considered what she needed for her upcoming trip to her husband's village outside of Kabwe, an old mining town just north of Lusaka. She had a singular purpose; she wanted to bring back a child who could help her with the cleaning, cooking, and laundry. The housework was too much for her now that both she and her husband were sick. His health had been deteriorating for months prior to his TB and HIV diagnoses, and the frequency with which he suffered periods of debilitation had increased. Mrs. Simwonde, too, was sick, but with diabetes and high blood pressure. Her doctor told her that these diagnoses were a result of the weight she had put on over the years and her love of salt. The medicines available in George never worked for her, and she could not afford the higher cost medications available elsewhere. She met the doctor's suggestion to lose weight with incredulity. How would it look for her to lose weight at a time when her husband was so sick? People would begin to talk about their increasing poverty. Her weight loss would further confirm people's suspicions about her husband's diagnosis and her own possible HIV seropositivity.

Mrs. Simwonde needed help in the household that only a child could offer, given the flexibility children had in their living arrangements—a flexibility that older people did not have. Her seventeen- and eleven-year-old sons were helping more since both she and Mr. Simwonde had become sick. But they could not accomplish everything that needed to get done. Her older son had school that kept him away all day. Her younger son, Mulenga, assisted with chores, but Mrs. Simwonde did not expect or want him to do everything. He still needed to focus on school if he was to support the family when he was older.

The creases in Mrs. Simwonde's face deepened as she assessed the gifts she would need to bring to the village for her visit. She had not been there for years and wanted to show goodwill to her husband's kin, and gifts would show that

they were doing well in Lusaka (even if they were not). Mrs. Simwonde was to
enact the class differences typically involved in receiving children.[10] Her gifts
would signify the household's ability to provide for a child entrusted to their care.
Guardians would not want a child to go so far away without some assurance that
the child would derive benefits from the move. As Maureen suggested in her jesting, there were reciprocal expectations when a child moved in and accomplished
domestic work. However, these were not always upheld, and deciding whom to
trust with one's children was a difficult endeavor.

A couple weeks after she left, Mrs. Simwonde returned on a bus with twelve-
year-old Ruth by her side. Though Ruth had always lived in rural villages, she
navigated life in the Simwondes' household and in George with ease. She carried
out household chores alongside Mrs. Simwonde and Mulenga and got along well
with both. With Ruth in the house, Mrs. Simwonde had time to rest and her skin
looked brighter than it had in a long time. Still, Mrs. Simwonde rejected the idea
that Ruth was there only to work. She said that she considered her a daughter and
began looking for schools in the area.

People took notice of the changes to the household since Ruth's arrival and,
one afternoon not too long after Ruth arrived, an older man visited the household to tell Mr. Simwonde that he would like Ruth to come live with him. Mr. and
Mrs. Simwonde were not prepared for such a suggestion. The man strengthened
his argument by drawing on notions of matrilineal descent, or matriliny. In a
matrilineal system, mothers and maternal relatives bear primary responsibility
for children, and children tend to form closer affective and material ties to maternal relatives. Ruth, he pointed out, was related to Mr. Simwonde through her
father's side. However, Ruth and he were related through Ruth's mother, making
his relation to Ruth stronger than theirs. Descent has long been seen to structure
kin obligations, and most groups in George might be considered as matrilineal, rather than patrilineal, where descent is traced through a father. The reality
that Ruth came to live with the Simwonde family demonstrates that matriliny
is neither inflexible nor deterministic.[11] However, the man's matrilineal relatedness provided compelling evidence of his greater rights to and responsibility for
Ruth. Though he had not gone to Kabwe to meet with Ruth's guardians and had
not sought their approval, as Mrs. Simwonde had, the idiom of matriliny proved
enough to dissuade the Simwondes from disagreeing with the move, at least too
outwardly. Ruth moved into the man's house, with the Simwondes expressing
their annoyance in private.

Mrs. Simwonde said it was a mistake to bring Ruth from Kabwe, but she had
wanted to avoid the longer, more expensive, and arduous trip to her own village in
Northern Province. Now, though, she was without an alternative. Mr. Simwonde's
eldest son, who lived elsewhere in Lusaka, gave her the money to go to her village.
She returned with thirteen-year-old Veronica, and Veronica, like Ruth, became

part of the rhythm of day-to-day life in the household. Mrs. Simwonde began look-ing into school placements, again, this time for Veronica. However, shortly after Veronica arrived, Mr. Simwonde stopped working, the household's money dwin-dled, and Mrs. Simwonde's promise to send Veronica to school went unfulfilled.

Veronica was expected to do more household chores than the Simwondes' sons, but she was not, otherwise, treated so differently. The older son stopped his schooling during this same time because the family could no longer afford the school fees associated with secondary school, and they needed the money he earned from piecework for their more basic needs, rather than to be used for schooling. Mulenga, their youngest son, remained in a no-fee government primary school, though not without his own struggles to meet the multiple costs associated with free schooling. He convinced his oldest brother, who lived out-side of George, to help him purchase a new uniform and shoes. He also per-suaded me to help out, catching me when we were out of earshot of his parents to ask that I buy him pencils and notebooks. The things that put Mulenga at an advantage over Veronica in terms of going to school were his social connections outside of the household and the fact that he was already enrolled in school.

Illness and poverty were a part of the Simwondes' family life, as they were for most, if not all, families in George and many families in other areas of sub-Saharan Africa that are heavily affected by HIV. The Simwondes were not unique in their reliance on children or the difficulties they encountered in providing for children in their household. What the Simwondes' experience shows most directly is that households were constantly changing in terms of resources, health, and membership. Such flux meant that the benefits and difficulties of keeping children constantly shift. Adults and, as we will later see, children must readjust to this shifting terrain with a view to both short-term needs and longer-term goals.

Keeping One's Own Children

Part of my survey of 200 households in George focused on where and with whom children lived. My snapshot of these households identified that children between the ages of six and fourteen lived in large households with many different rela-tives. The majority of children (77 percent) reportedly lived with their mothers, among other relatives. Fewer children lived with both their mothers and fathers (54 percent) or with only their fathers (4 percent). When children did not reside in households with either a mother or a father (among other kin), they most fre-quently lived with maternal grandparents or other maternal relatives, primarily sisters and brothers of their mother. The percentages above cannot adequately capture the variability of children's living arrangements. In Zambia, the notion of family is wide and can be extended indefinitely through categories such as mother, father, grandparent, sister, brother, uncle, and so forth (Colson 1958). For example, a mother's sister can be a mother. Similarly, a distant cousin can be referred to as sister or brother. These data, then, may not necessarily suggest a discrete biological connection but rather a social one.

Knowing with whom children were living can provide some information on adults' responsibilities and rights to children. However, understanding where and why children move provides insight into the more active process of how people grappled with their rights and responsibilities to children. Based on my observations in George and the previous literature in Zambia, I had expected to identify a lot of circulation among the children in the surveyed households. Rather than validating my assumptions about the degree to which children circulated among households, however, respondents emphasized children's lack of movement. Many children in the surveyed households (85 percent of the 313 children) were reported to have lived with the surveyed household since birth, without ever making an unaccompanied move.[12]

Keeping one's own child—even if that child was not a biological child, but a grandchild or sibling's child—was an expectation of good guardianship. "Nowadays things are difficult," one man told me in response to my questions about whether children had moved in or out of his house, "so you can't send your children." He and other respondents told cautionary tales about why they could not send children to live in relatives' homes. Sending a child was seen as a last resort, something that reflected poorly on a guardian. As with the Simwondes' case, you never know how the living situation in the household might change and affect the child or other people in the household. Sending children away from home was seen as a violation of parental responsibility that reflected on the parent and could have implications for relationships between households and generations.

While keeping one's own children was seen as a marker of good guardianship, not receiving and taking care of relatives' children exposed a household's financial hardship. One man answering my survey clarified why no children had moved into his household with the statement: "I am failing to look after my children. Why should I let other people's children suffer [like my children do]?" Other respondents suggested that they would like to keep relatives' children, but the children's guardians would not send them, and the children did not want to come. When considering why children were not coming to live in her household, one woman suggested: "Maybe because we are not working. But before [my husband] stopped work, we used to live with a lot of [child] relatives." The circulation of children has been seen as an important survival strategy for poor households in Zambia and beyond, but the responses I received suggested that keeping children was both an expense and a resource that poor people were finding harder to afford.[13]

Part of this emphasis on caring for one's own child reflected the discourses of development initiatives that are advancing Euro-American ideals of parenthood, the nuclear family, and child vulnerability.[14] However, ideals about shared rights to children remained, even if they were upheld in discussions of breach when adults expressed nostalgia and regret about not being able to keep children because of poverty.[15] I do not view such responses as suggestive of the increasing insularity of households. Children's lack of movement may have been, in part, an effort to keep family relationships intact by not overburdening kin or causing children to suffer. In chapter 5, I will show how such avoidances became a strategy to cultivate shared familial responsibilities and obligations to a child when her mother became sick.

Despite the survey respondents' explicit emphasis on the sedentariness of children, there was much evidence of children's circulation. Out of 313 children ages six to fourteen in the surveyed households, 47 children (15 percent) moved into the households of kin at some point in their lives. Of these children, most came to the household after the death of a parent or other guardian (23 children) or as a result of other forms of hardship, such as illness, marital problems, and food shortages, in their previous households (12 children). The remaining children moved in to help with chores or childcare (4 children), receive schooling (3 children), or just because the child or someone in the household wanted to live together (5 children).[16]

There were also 44 children—not counted among the 313 children currently living in the households—who had moved out of the 200 surveyed households during the two years prior to my survey. Most of these children were temporary household residents, who had come in because of crises (mostly the death of a guardian) and who left because the household was "suffering too much," another relative wanted to live with the child, or the child wanted to leave. The responses to my survey suggest that adults continued to enact shared responsibilities for children, but that, most frequently, extreme crisis propelled such children's movements into and out of households.

Beyond the survey, my observations in Zambia over more than a decade led me to suspect that there was even more circulation than the survey revealed. Adults were going to great lengths to foster belonging for children in their households, through "forgetting" children's moves, both on the survey and in everyday conversations. I witnessed this in the households I followed for more than a year when I belatedly learned about a child's parentage or their earlier moves. My observations match those of other researchers in sub-Saharan Africa, who have noted adults' efforts to protect children through reframing children's relationships and compelling children to forget their first homes (Archambault 2010, Ross 2010). A number of factors shape adults' reasons for forgetting children's moves, among these are the global discourses advanced by humanitarian efforts aimed at AIDS orphans, which I will discuss in more detail in the following sections and from the children's points of view.

Children's Relationships in and across Households

The above material raises the question: How do children feel about their circulations and interpret their belonging to households when their moves were both necessary and difficult? I consider the cases of ten-year-old Abby Banda, whom I have introduced in the previous chapters, and twelve-year-old Musa Njovu to illustrate broader aspects of how children experienced and strategized where they were kept, from the points of view and the actions of the children. As both cases make evident, belonging to a household was about much more than accessing material resources or carrying out domestic work. It was about the relationships children were able to build or not within particular households, and what such relationships meant for their future life chances.

Abby

When I first met Abby, she was living in an uncle's house with her mother and siblings. Her uncle, an unmarried relative who worked as a bus conductor, spent long hours away from the house. Elesia, Abby's mother, and the children moved there one night after Abby's father had forced them out of his house. The reason he kicked them out, I was told, was that "he was tired of having a sick wife." Elesia had been sick on and off for years with what she considered recurrent meningitis. She suspected that she had meningitis again at the time they were forced from their home, though after moving into the relative's house, she found out that she had TB. As I described in the introduction, her diagnosis compelled her relatives to move Abby and her sister to the family house in a different part of George, to be cared for by another uncle, Elesia's brother. Elesia moved across Lusaka to receive care from her sister.

To understand how Abby understood her care during this time, I asked her to draw "all of the people who care for you" and "what they do to take care," an assignment I gave to all of the children. As with all of the drawings the children made, Abby and the other children produced varied depictions of their caregivers based on their past experiences and their day-to-day realities at the time of the drawing. They tailored their drawings to what they thought I might wish to see in such a drawing and also in response to the reactions they expected from other children and adults present during the exercise. In other words, the drawings were a lot like the verbal or written responses of research participants, young or old, to any interview questions; they were intersubjective (Toren 2007). These aspects do not reduce the value of children's drawings for understanding children's views on their own situations or the nature of familial care more generally. Instead, they make them particularly informative for illustrating not only the decisions children make about whom they consider caregivers and the places where they might receive good care, but also their interpretations of these decisions.

Using a pencil, Abby outlined four figures standing in a row. She drew an aunt first. An uncle stood next to her aunt and next to him stood the man with whom she was living at the time of the drawing, her mother's brother.[17] Last in the line was her mother. After outlining their bodies, she colored them in hues of brown, orange, yellow, and red. Her aunt was robust and wore nice clothing. She had her arm extended and a kwacha note in her hand. Her uncle also looked well off, though he held his hands by his side. Her mother's brother, with whom she lived, was very thin and wore the tattered trousers of a poor man. Her mother looked healthier than she appeared in real life, indicative of the way Abby wished her to be. Abby described each figure in turn:

> HER AUNT: "My aunt bought me a uniform, socks, a bag, and shoes when I was going to school. She asked me to live with her so she could send me to school."
>
> HER UNCLE: "This is my uncle. He told my mother that she should look for a school for me. If she finds a school, he will pay for it."
>
> HER MOTHER'S BROTHER (*in an annoyed tone*): "He keeps me and my sister. He only buys us food. Since we arrived, he has not bought us clothes."
>
> HER MOTHER: "My mother feeds me, buys me clothes, and cares for me."

When Abby made her drawing, she had not intended to depict her father, the man her mother had married when Abby was a baby. She added him only when Olivious mentioned that he was not pictured. She penciled him in as a stick figure and said she did not want to color him because he had a "bad heart." The entire time they lived together he either wanted her gone or treated her as hired help. He had never given her anything.

Abby's drawing and related discussion offer several clues into the ways in which the children conceptualized care. She made a distinction between "keeping" and "caring" that revealed both her expectations and resentments. The Nyanja word *kusunga* translates roughly as to keep, raise, bring up, or look after others. Kusunga is almost always used in reference to the activities that occur in houses. The word typically refers to children, but can also be used to describe keeping anyone who is perceived as a dependent, such as the sick, elderly, and even women. Children made distinctions between kusunga (to keep) and other words for care such as *kusamala* (to care or protect) and *kuthandiza* (to help). For example, someone might say: "*Andisunga ndi a Bwalya, koma sandisamala bwino* [the one who keeps me is Bwalya, but he does not take care of me properly]."[18]

When Abby spoke of her uncle as keeping but not caring for her, she was expressing resentment for unfulfilled expectations. I suspect that her statement was made in reference to the large burden of household work she had to accomplish at the time of the drawing and her fears about her future. At the bottom of her page of caregivers, she drew herself in three scenes. The first scene was her eating with her mother, and the second was her eating with her mother's brother. The last scene featured her eating together with her sister. Elesia's brother— pictured in the middle scene—had gone to great lengths to accommodate Abby and her sister, notably moving his own wife and children out of the house so that he could fulfill his obligations to his sister. However, at the time of the drawing, he spent most days trying to find work or carrying out piecework, making Abby carry out much of the household chores and care for her younger sister. She worried that she was gaining the identity of a domestic worker, and she expressed concerns about whether she would receive her education. These concerns came out clearly when her aunt asked Abby to move to her house so that she could send her to school. Abby was suspicious of her aunt's motives. She thought that she wanted her only for housework because she had proven herself to be a good worker in her uncle's house. She worried that her aunt might not honor her promise to send her to school.

In the children's terms, to care for a child, rather than simply keep them, means to advocate for their well-being. Abby and other children expressed that having an advocate in their household mattered. An advocate provides for the child, gathers resources from kin, and organizes a child's schooling and other needs. Advocates were people who had love for children and encouraged and taught them in ways that helped them grow to full personhood. Advocates were interested in a child's future and warded off ill-meaning kin who might wish to take the child into their households because of their ability to accomplish domestic work, without consideration of the child's needs. A child might have advocates in a couple of houses and move between them, as a couple of children showed when they linked houses together in their drawings on topics of family and also of care.

Children depended on adults for many things, including growth toward social personhood,[19] and this dependence figured into how children viewed adults' dependence on them. Abby and the other children made key distinctions between activities they did for adults that they considered as "work" versus "help." These distinctions did not hang on the type or amount of work but upon the relationship between themselves and the persons for whom they carried out chores or other activities. Instead, "work" referred to domestic and other productive activities carried out for people who did not care for them materially or affectively, and did not help them grow toward adulthood. "Help" was domestic work and other productive activities that the children felt were reciprocated. The distinctions they made related to what they received from adults that helped them in the present, but most especially into the future. These included an adult's love, loyalty, and encouragement as well as their ability to facilitate a child's schooling and access resources such as clothing and food.

Even though many people could and did serve as advocates, Abby and other children emphasized the role of the (social or biological) mother. This suggests specific concerns about what might happen to their well-being in the absence of a mother or mother-like figure. Their concerns reminded me of the adults who spoke of the need to care for one's own children. Further, as I will show in later sections, their concerns touched on ideals of parenting that were emerging within the current political economic context in Zambia and also within a humanitarian context that has emphasized the plights of orphans.

Musa

In May 2008, Musa Njovu's mother, Judy, received two calls from relatives living on the Copperbelt. The first call was from a newly married couple with well-paying jobs and a newborn baby. They wanted twelve-year-old Musa to come live with them. They asked that he help out with the baby and housework and, in return, they promised to send him to a good private school. Their decision to ask Musa, rather than other child relatives, to move to their house was most likely shaped by the extreme situation in Judy's household that would make the opportunity both attractive and difficult to decline. For months the members of Judy's household had barely made ends meet. Exacerbating the strain on the household, Judy was beginning to suffer extreme joint pain. The second call that Judy received was from her oldest daughter's husband, who also lived in the same city on the Copperbelt. Hilda, Musa's sister, was critically ill, and Hilda's husband was overwhelmed by the severity of her illness and her nursing needs. He needed Judy to help with her medical appointments and nursing care. This latter call meant that there would be no hedging about Musa's move. With Judy leaving, the household had few other choices: Musa would move in with his newly wed relatives.

"Are you excited about going to a private school?" I asked Musa the day before he left for the Copperbelt with his mother. Musa shrugged in a way that made it hard to tell if he was excited, resigned, or just thought my question was odd. After all, it did not seem that he had much choice in the matter. His mother also seemed resigned, repeating that Musa's best chance for a good education was away from George. Since Musa's older brother had died the year before from TB and other complications due to AIDS, Musa had taken on many of the household responsibilities. His mother, who was still distraught from her son's death, spent most of her time at church, receiving financial, emotional, and spiritual assistance from fellow church members. Musa's two older brothers and his younger brother were busy in school. They spent most of their days away from home.

Musa was usually the only one home during my visits, and he was often carrying out chores or studying on his own when I came.

I am still unsure about Musa's parentage. When I asked his older brother once why he did not help Musa with the household chores, he told me that Musa was the son of a deceased man who had not married Judy. At the time, this seemed like a peculiar response to an outwardly unrelated question. It was something that Judy never admitted, saying that Musa's father was the same man who fathered her older children. He too had died years ago. Musa's younger brother, Mumba, had a different father who not only acknowledged Mumba but also gave Judy money to pay for his private schooling. What seemed obvious was that Musa was unable to draw on the resources of other adults as freely as Judy's other children. When chores needed to be done, they fell on Musa, leaving a number of observers in the neighborhood commenting that Musa was "the woman of the house." I heard this phrase spoken about boys and girls (including Abby) at other times in my research when children took on the bulk of the housework. It not only pointed to the gender construction of housework in Zambia but also indexed boys' and girls' undirected (by an adult) and excessive housework as out of place.

There were two aspects of Musa's schooling and education that made him more available for housework than his brothers. He was in fourth grade at the nearby government school where he had not yet learned to read and write and his school day lasted roughly three hours. His older brothers had received private school educations when they were young and their father was still alive. Musa began his schooling after this father had already died. In the eyes of his older brothers, the facts of his illiteracy made his primary schooling less important than their secondary schooling and the all-day private schooling of his eight-year-old brother. The reality that Musa's school days were so short also meant that Musa had much more free time than anyone else in the household. In other words, a number of factors combined to make him the least materially supported member of the household. His mother worried about this and viewed the move to the Copperbelt as an opportunity for Musa to receive a good education.

With borrowed money, Judy bought Musa new clothes for the journey, and they set out on a bus together. After staying only four days in the house of the newly wed relatives, Musa ran away. He found his chance to leave when his "sister" (Musa's term) took her baby to the market in search of school shoes for Musa. She returned with shoes in hand to an empty house and frantically called Judy to let her know that Musa was missing. Judy set out along the road to the relatives' house, attempting to cover the ground that Musa might walk. When she could not find him, she went back to her sick daughter's house and waited. Just before dark, Musa showed up, surprising everyone with his ability to navigate the streets on his own. The effort he went to leave the house made the family reconsider his move and, several days later, Judy returned to Lusaka on a bus, with both Musa and her ailing daughter by her side.

I headed straight to Musa's house when I heard he had returned to George. We sat together on a couch. I asked trivial questions about his trip: What was the house like? What did you think of their new baby? Was she a good baby? Finally, I worked up the courage to ask why he had run away. He said: "Me, I can't stay without my mother. I am used [to staying with her]. I have been staying with my mother my whole life, and suddenly I start staying with my sister. It was very difficult for me so I decided to come back." I asked what he would have done if his mother had refused to take him back or the newly wed relatives had refused to let him go. He said that he would have waited until the end of the school term, at which time he would ask to visit his mother in Lusaka and then, during his visit to Lusaka, refuse to return to the Copperbelt.

To justify his decisions to his family and me, Musa drew on child protection discourses that focus on orphans, but with a twist because his mother was still alive. Mothers, he argued, rather than other relatives, love a child enough to give them proper care. If a mother is alive, other relatives will always wonder why she has chased her child from her home. A child who is chased from home becomes just like an orphan. In Musa's account, social orphanhood could unleash a chain of negative events. Relatives and other community members would use the rejection as an excuse to neglect the child, make him work, or send him to the streets. Parental death offered a ready explanation as to why relatives should care; being cast away by a living parent did not. There was something about a child moving in the absence of parental death that indexed a larger problem with the household, the child, or the parents.

In Kristen Cheney's (2007) research in Uganda, she has shown that children draw on the language of international child rights discourses on issues such as schooling and abuse to justify the difficult decisions they make. Such discourses, she suggested, could shape children's actions and hopes as well as add to their anxieties when children were powerless to change their situations. Musa's defense of his move back to his mother's house provides yet another example of how children interpret and repurpose global discourses within the contexts of their lives. Musa made a connection between his circumstances and that of orphans, who have become a main global humanitarian category in southern Africa in the HIV era. The importance of examining how children incorporate such discourses into their understandings of kin relationships was brought home to me throughout Abby's emphasis on advocating kin and Musa's emphasis on living with his mother.

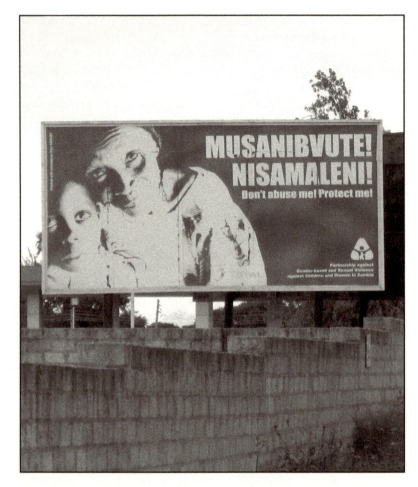

Fig. 2.1 Billboard in Kalingalinga in 2008, an example of the child protection messages that were part of the built landscape. A child's voice commands adults to protect, rather than abuse, children. The billboard does not make explicit the orphan status of the child, but the grandmother figure gives the impression that the child's parents were not present in the child's life. Photo by Nicholas Kahn-Fogel.

GLOBAL DISCOURSES OF CHILDREN'S RESIDENCE
AND RELATIONSHIPS: THE ORPHAN

Since the early years of the HIV epidemic, the orphan, defined as a child who has lost one or both parents,[20] has been viewed as the quintessential vulnerable child.[21] The discourses around orphans are powerful and come from diverse sources: the media, international NGOs, government officials, and school lessons, to name a few. However, despite the diversity of sources, the stories about orphans can follow a fixed trajectory, giving the reader a feeling of déjà vu with each reading. South African researchers Helen Meintjes and Sonja Geise (2006) have named this trajectory the "orphan mythology." Such accounts move implicitly—and sometimes explicitly—from notions of parental death to other risks, such as life on the street, physical or sexual abuse, excessive labor, and school dropout. For example, Meintjes and Geise described a 2003 United Nations Children's Emergency Fund (UNICEF) report on orphans and vulnerable children in Zambia that made the claim that most street children in Lusaka were orphans. In fact, as Meintjes and Geise (2006) pointed out, 78 percent of children cited in the report actually had a living parent. As they argued, policies and programs in southern Africa have been so preoccupied with the absence of families and deaths of parents that they have ignored the presence of adults, including living parents. The orphan discourse is, thus, all about children's residence and their family relationships, though often in absentia.

Though that 2003 UNICEF report is now quite old and there is a general sense among the humanitarian workers I know that the term orphan can be stigmatizing, such claims have continued. These claims are used to draw attention to very real poverty and suffering and, importantly, compel funders to action. Take for example the comments of Edgar Lungu—Zambia's president as of this writing (then minister of home affairs)—in 2013, after visiting Misisi, an area of Lusaka that is similar to George in its economic marginalization and burden of HIV and TB. In a *Lusaka Voice* article on December 23, 2013, Lungu was reported to have said: "The serious consequences of HIV and AIDS and tuberculosis in Misisi have subjected many children to misery, leaving them with no hope for a better future, hence they end up on the streets . . . This in turn increases the burden on society. The number of street kids in Misisi keeps rising by the day, which also leaves the girl child with no option but to be forced into sex work for survival." While he avoided mentioning orphans, the category was very much implied as the consequence of HIV and TB.

Children were familiar with the large media and programmatic focus on orphans, especially the particular mythology about the trajectory of children from loving, stable homes to abusive homes or to life on the street (see fig. 2.1). The pervasiveness of these discourses became especially evident during almost all of the children's tape-recorded storytelling. I had given every child drawings to use during their recorded storytelling, including two different drawings of children seated alone. Speaking into the tape recorders, most children referred to the children in the drawings as orphans. Some related the drawings to their own experiences, and many offered accounts of what happens to orphans—"they later become street children"—or they made more general pleas for mothers to care for orphans.

Take for example the recording made by ten-year-old Sarafina, who spoke in English to convey the lesson in her recording. The children rarely spoke in

English and typically only to repeat lessons, songs, or poems learned in school. To make the recording, Sarafina went outside of her house and called on her younger neighbor to participate:

> SARAFINA: If there is a child without parents, she will always stay alone. Some are always crying because a lot are beaten in the streets. We see them. Some don't even go to school. We see them playing around the compound. So we should be keeping orphans. Please we beg you mothers, we should help them in any form of help. Please, mothers, we beg you.
>
> SARAFINA: [To her neighbor] Repeat after me. If in your area there are orphans we should be keeping them.
>
> NEIGHBOR: If in your area there are orphans we should be keeping them.
>
> SARAFINA: You should be buying clothes for them and food.
>
> NEIGHBOR: You should be buying clothes for them and food.
>
> SARAFINA: We must cooperate to help them so we beg you mothers to take care of orphans.
>
> NEIGHBOR: We must cooperate to help them so we beg you mothers to take care of orphans.
>
> SARAFINA: And even clothes and food are important. Please please mothers, we beg you. So we are asking our mothers to cooperate with others in helping orphans.
>
> NEIGHBOR: And even clothes and food are important. Please please mothers, we beg you. So we are asking our mothers to cooperate with others in helping orphans.
>
> SARAFINA: We beg you our mothers. Okay, let's get in [the house].

The focus on mothers is accentuated in Sarafina's exposition about orphans in a way that calls forth broader notions of the responsibility of mothers, which Musa also referred to and which I discuss in detail in chapter 5.

Twelve-year-old Samson also focused on women's responsibility to protect children in his response to one of the drawings. Speaking for the girl in the drawing, he said: "'I need help because I don't have a mother.'" He continued to explain: "She gets no response from the people near her. This girl needs help like accommodation, protection, and food." In both Sarafina's and Samson's accounts, the children needed help because they did not have a social or biological mother. Still further, they suggested a failure of kinship care that necessitated a broader community response to helping children. They called for new mothers to step in, though it is unclear if such mothers do. In Samson's words, "She gets no response."

Abby drew on similar understandings of orphans to interpret the events in her life and express fears about her future. She began her story by saying, "Here I see the child crying." She continued:

Her mother died. When your mother dies, even if your aunt takes very good care of you, still you will have memories of the times you spent with your mother. Death is very bad. That's why this girl is crying. Even me, it would hurt me very badly if my mother had died when she was sick with TB. Who would take care of me? As to my side, I always pray to God to let my mother take care of me at least up to a stage where I can take care of myself and do the same to my sister and my brother. Not her dying, leaving me at this stage. No! No! Because some aunts say: "They are orphans, I will do whatever I want to do with them." That's what happens to orphans. They later become street kids. No one can forget his or her mother!

Her orphan narrative focused on the possibility of her own mother's death and the fear that she might have no one to care for her. She described the process of forgetting one's first mother as fraught because relatives might not allow such forgetting when they treat children as orphans.

Abby described a key aspect of the children's understandings of orphanhood: orphanhood occurred through familial and social rejection: "Some aunts say: 'They are orphans, I will do whatever I want to do with them.' That's what happens to orphans. They later become street kids." Becoming an orphan related to the death of her mother, but it was more so about the loss of nurture and protection from relatives in a mother's absence. In the previous section, Musa demonstrated that death does not have to occur for a child to become an orphan. A move away from a mother figure or person who advocated for a child could make a child an orphan. An orphan was, thus, not a static category defined by parental death, but a fluid category that children could move into and out of, depending upon their place of residence as well as the quality and social perceptions of their relationships. An orphan was a child who was cast away, uncared for, and unloved. The term marked a child who had been removed from recognizable forms of sociality in which adults—primarily women as mothers—gave care and love to children. The children tried hard to avoid orphanhood through nurturing specific relationships and remaining in or trying to get back to specific places. It is notable that, according to international standards, Abby, Musa, Samson, and Sarafina were already "orphans" given that each child had experienced the death of one biological parent. But this was not an identity that they claimed for themselves and neither did seven other children in my study whose biological mothers or fathers had died.

To emphasize the importance of the children's statements and my points, I return to Meintjes and Geise's critique of the 2003 UNICEF report that suggested that most street children were orphans. They argued that if implying that most street children in Lusaka are orphans "is a decisive rhetorical strategy to bring attention to a desperate situation, we are troubled by the inflammation of the orphan mythology, for in longer terms this is a powerful and counterproductive form of othering" (2006, 411). My observations suggest that Meintjes and Geise's longer-term projection was materializing in George. Children were resisting such othering through their residential and relationship choices and also using it to inform their fears about the future when such choices were out of their control.

"Going on Holiday": Moves That Do Not Stigmatize

Children did not react to all moves away from their usual homes with resistance and trepidation. Sometimes children desired to leave the places where they lived or that they considered home. In this section, I discuss a type of circulation that the children spoke about with anticipation and excitement. It is a form of shorter-term circulation among households in which children engage in Zambia and other parts of sub-Saharan Africa. This movement is so mundane and ostensibly happy that it has gone virtually unnoticed within concerns about children's movements in crisis. As I will show, it is nevertheless important for understanding kinship care for children who live in areas affected by illness, death, and poverty. This practice is called "going on holiday."[22]

In Zambia, the word holiday—spoken in English—refers to school breaks. Schools have three month-long holidays—one in August before the start of the new school year, one during Christmastime, and another in April. Each break represents an opportunity for a ritualized form of movement from children's usual homes to the homes of relatives. Far from trivial, shorter-term movements may serve as critical moments to nurture reciprocity and care between households and also make and unmake particular kinds of childhoods.

On a chilly July morning in 2008, I finished sweeping a layer of brown dust out of the demonstration building on the grounds of the government health center in George. The building was one large room—typically reserved for storage and lined with bicycles and wheelbarrows donated for health projects. That day, I was conducting one of several workshops with the children. We started the day with a group discussion, which I had developed into a game. The object of the game was simple. I had made a large foam die with pictures of different topics pasted on each side. The children took turns throwing the die and drawing questions from brown paper sacks that corresponded with the side on which they landed.

Despite the playfulness of the method, the tone of our discussion was serious. The children outlined why and when children move households and talked more deeply about the ramifications of movement. They spoke of death as one of the only times when a child would move away from her home. They used terms such as "orphan" and "street child" and connected movements with isolation, a lack of care and love, homelessness, abuse, and exploitation.

But then the tenor of the discussion took a dramatic turn. Here's what happened: Mulenga passed the foam die to Annie. She threw it in the air; it bounced off a bench and landed on a drawing of two houses connected by a path. This was an image many of the children had drawn during my visits to their homes to indicate connections between households. Reaching into the accompanying bag, Annie pulled out the question: "What is holiday?" Chatter filled the room. Several children jumped out of their seats.

Holiday was exciting. Speaking in Nyanja, Annie explained, "Holiday is when you tell your mother that you want to visit relatives when you close school. Maybe you get escorted by an elder sibling. And when school opens, you come back." The type of movement Annie described was so common among the children in my study that nearly half of them were away from their homes during each school holiday. In the larger survey I conducted among 200 households, I found that 71 out of 313 children ages six to fourteen years old had gone on holiday during the last school break, roughly 23 percent of the sample.[23] While this number is less dramatic than my observations during the long-term household study, it still shows a substantial amount of movement during school holidays.

The children waited for Annie to answer the question about holiday, then they spoke over one another to describe the contours of holiday. It was hard to overlook the pride, excitement, and anticipation generated by my holiday questions (see fig. 2.2). The children described the aesthetic pleasure of holiday. Holidays were for socializing with relatives they rarely saw, listening to music, dancing, and participating in celebrations. Ten-year-old Rita captured this aesthetic pleasure in a pencil drawing she gave me upon her return from a holiday spent at her granny's house. The drawing included relatives who came for a Christmas party. When describing the drawing to me, she pointed to a radio: They had listened to traditional Zambian music and danced, she told me.

Part of the aesthetics of holiday revolved around the food and gifts that the children received from relatives. In Zambia, as Henrietta Moore and Megan Vaughan (1994) have shown, the provision of clothing and food has long made tangible the social relations across households and contributed to the fulfillment of obligations. Children emphasized that holidays were not just times to attain clothing and other needs; they were times to attain *school* clothing and needs. As I have shown, the children strongly associated school with their current and future well-being. Even small contributions toward their schooling held tremendous symbolic value, representing a relative's investment in their future. The children's drawings of the people who cared for them shifted substantially after their return from holidays as the children highlighted relatives who lived across or outside of Lusaka, rather than the household members who were typically depicted in such drawings.

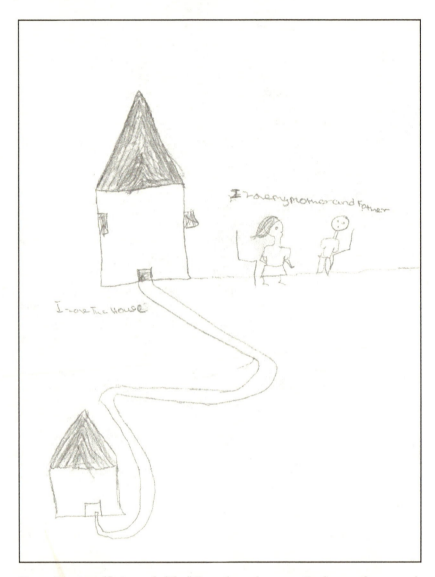

Fig. 2.2 Drawing of "going on holiday." Tracy shows the connection between her parents' and grandparents' houses, which became evident during her holiday visits with her grandparents. Tracy wrote, "I love my mother and father" and "I love the house," in reference to her grandparents and their house. Drawing by Tracy, age twelve.

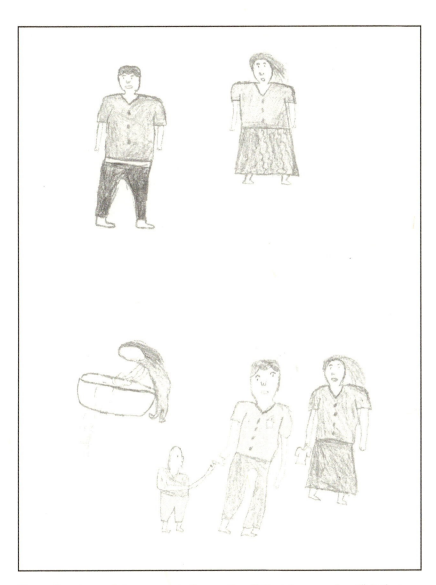

Fig. 2.3 Drawing made in response to the question: "Who takes care of you?" At the top, Stephen drew his uncle (father's sister's husband) and his aunt (mother's sister), who live in different parts of Lusaka. Underneath, he drew his aunt washing clothes for him while he visited her during holiday. He also drew his uncle giving him money during a holiday visit and his uncle's wife (his father's sister) giving him clothes that she had bought for him. Drawing by Stephen, age eleven.

Holidays were not, however, primarily about money and financial support for children. The children expected to become embedded in the division of labor in the households. As Eness explained: "When they go for work, you sweep their house and wash plates." The children highlighted that holidays were times to contribute to the care of grandparents, newborn babies, or sick relatives. They indicated the importance of such caring and domestic activities and took pride in their ability to contribute.

In describing the many aspects of holiday, children were referencing a particular locus of care that extends across households. It was a locus of care in which they participated and benefited and in which they played important roles. With kin spread across residential areas in Lusaka, holidays provided a time for children to nurture relationships in multiple households—their usual households and the households they visited—while remaining in school and not overwhelming kin or moving away from their preferred home. It may not be too far of a reach to suggest that such work across households and within shortened time frames contributed to the survival of some households. Regardless of their impact on survival, holidays served as attempts to forge forms of sociality that, in Patricia Henderson's words, "looked to the future, but that were deeply imbricated with repertoires that had some continuity with the past" (2013, 14). While Henderson was writing of the maintenance of marriage rituals in South Africa's HIV epidemic, holidays were also a sort of social occasion. By setting the children up as school-going, contributing, and cared-for children, this social occasion strongly resisted discourses about child isolation, abandonment, and family breakdown, which I described in the previous sections of this chapter.

Holiday presented a time when constructs such as kinship and home were mobilized to naturalize and also call into question social divisions, categories, and identities (Ngwane 2003). As I will show later in chapter 5, a child's holiday movement to a relative's house helped maintain the appearance of a normative childhood for a girl whose mother was ill. In another household, a child's holiday movement offered a sick woman the help she needed to maintain her house and marriage.

Holidays could also naturalize differences, such as the difference between school-going children and out-of-school children, relatively well-off and poorer households, and children with nearer or farther away family members. Particular children were more desired as holiday visitors than others. This followed along various lines of difference among children and households, with some children desired for either their ability to contribute labor or their school-going status and potential for success.

As a normative form of movement, holiday offered an opening for a number of processes and practices that could not happen at other times of the year without causing social disruptions. Some parents and guardians worried about the motives of relatives, who might wish to keep a child after the holiday ended. One woman explained to me that she did not allow her granddaughter to go on holiday because it meant she would leave school permanently. She believed that relatives would become accustomed to her granddaughter's productive contributions in their household, viewing her more like an orphan than a daughter. Her suspicions proved partially correct during a later school holiday when her granddaughter left for holiday and did not return to her household or to school. However, complicating ideas about who orchestrated that move, children in the girl's neighborhood told me that the girl had wished to move out of her grandmother's house for the longer term and stay with the relatives she was visiting. I observed other children orchestrate moves away from their households under the guise of going on holiday. Musa told me he, too, would have moved back to his mother's house during a school holiday and refused to return to the relatives' house on the Copperbelt. In this way, children considered holiday as a time to assert some control over their residential status and try out life in a different household, without damaging relationships or identities.

Conclusion

I began this chapter with a singular objective: to identify how children and adults were attempting to secure and enact good care for children at a time when HIV has affected many families and when households face chronic resource shortages. The fact that children as young as the children who took part in my study were not supporting themselves may seem obvious to readers. Yet this chapter should also make clear that children play an important role in the domestic economy, even when their actions are supportive of and initiated by adults (as opposed to self-guided and independent).[24] As I have shown, neither dependence nor independence fits what it meant to be a cared-for child in George. Instead, children and adults were dependent upon one another; they were interdependent.

In George, and likely many other places around the world, it is impossible to divorce what children do from what they receive and, yet, scholarly and policy discussions tend to separate children's doing from their receiving. Putting these two together—what children do and what they receive—can help us understand children's strategies and fears. For example, Pamela Reynolds has written about children's economic contributions and strategies in Zimbabwe. She suggested that, through both small and large activities carried out for adults, children in the rural area where she worked developed strategies to nurture specific kin relationships (1991, 77). My work has shown that children viewed such nurturing of relationships as instrumental to receiving the many things they needed in order to grow into social adulthood. Not all kin relationships were viewed the same, and children attempted to direct their productive activities toward the relationships that mattered to them. This depended upon their residence, which offered them proximity to people who advocated for them in many ways.

When talking about children's family care in George, it was impossible to ignore children's circulations and also the lengths to which children and adults went to keep children in place. The adults I surveyed underscored changes in children's circulation due to the poverty they and their families faced. Everyone, they said, must take care of their own children. Their emphasis on children staying in place may indicate that people were ascribing to a much more rigid concept of parenthood and home than typically described in previous studies on child circulation in sub-Saharan Africa (Archambault 2010). And yet, my survey suggests that children were still moving to help and be helped by adults, and adults were upholding strong values associated with caring for kin.

The children I knew were aware that residence in certain households, with certain people, could shape their identities and future prospects. They expressed that the key to long-term well-being was the ability to remain in the care of specific people who affirmed their identities and advocated for them. Moving to or living in particular places denied them such identities and relationships, or at least raised concerns about such a denial. A notable force in Zambia has been the large amount of attention and funding set aside for orphans, children whose parent or parents have died from HIV. Orphans have remained a consistent focus of international HIV relief funding, even though variables such as poverty prove more indicative of a child's needs than whether or not their parents are alive.[25] Children drew on the particular orphan mythology that has arisen to draw attention to children's needs—the mythology that orphanhood is equated to life on the streets, abuse, school dropout, and neglect. In their experiences, an orphan was not, however, defined by death of a biological parent, but by rejection. The mythology presented a grim picture of what it meant for their life chances when they moved away from adults who might advocate for them, particularly mothers, or when such moves appeared imminent because of illness.

Not all moves away from their households were so negatively evaluated. Holiday visits were less permanent and served as a creative attempt to nurture kin relations, reinforce particular valued identities, and exchange labor and resources in ways that current contexts and discourses make difficult. Holidays drew on conventional understandings of the circulation of children, but without the strains on households or stigma of circulations in which crisis is directly implicated. In its idealized form, going on holiday reinforced broader conceptualizations of the meaning of a good childhood in George. This included an emphasis on schooling, children's domestic contributions, and adult loyalty and affection. It offered a version of shared intergenerational and inter-household responsibility writ small that contrasted with, but was also deeply responsive to, ideas about children's detrimental movements within the context of HIV.

In this chapter, I described a range of ways in which children and adults constructed ideals about good care. I demonstrated that the chronicity of poor health and poverty and the prominence of global health initiatives shaped ideals about and practices of good care, as well as the interdependence between adults and children. I view this chapter as a foundation for the remaining chapters, in which I will demonstrate, still further, how proximity and the nurturing of particular relationships in specific places—what I referred to in the introduction as "being closer"—served as a strategy that the children turned to when guardians became ill.

CHAPTER 3

Between Silence and Disclosure

The deep lines in Mr. Simwonde's face make him look at once distinguished and tired. We met for the first time in August 2007 at George Health Centre after a nurse told him that his sputum smear tests were positive for TB. I watched their exchange from across the room. The nurse handed Mr. Simwonde medication for his first week of treatment and told him how to take it. When she finished explaining the medication, she asked if he had any children living in his home. He said that he had an eleven-year-old son named Mulenga, to which she pointed to where I sat and mentioned my study. Learning that my research was about children's care for their parents or guardians, Mr. Simwonde said that Mulenga was very caring, and he had become even more so during the previous months as Mr. Simwonde had become increasingly debilitated, due to TB and other infections. Mr. Simwonde later invited me to his home to meet both Mulenga and his wife, Mrs. Simwonde.

When I arrived at the family's home the following morning, Mr. Simwonde rushed Mulenga outside to play. He wanted me to tell him more about my study, my methods, and what I would do with my findings, and he wanted to read through the project description and informed consent forms. After our conversation, he gave me permission to ask Mulenga if he would like to participate in the study. But before he called Mulenga in from outdoors, he had one request: "Amake Mulenga [mother of Mulenga] and I are not telling Mulenga that I am sick with TB. We say it is malaria." His statement implied that I, too, should remain quiet about his specific diagnosis.

As I continued recruitment for that part of my study, I learned that few adults I spoke with had told their children about their TB diagnosis, and no adults diagnosed with HIV had directly mentioned HIV to their children. They concealed their HIV and TB diagnoses, they said, to protect and nurture their children. As

Mr. Simwonde told me, knowledge of TB might "disturb a child" and make him "think too much" about the illness and death of a guardian and, in turn, about the child's own current and future well-being. In the views of the guardians I spoke with, naming TB was harmful. It could break down relations between genera-tions and inhibit the process of building a child toward adulthood.

Though little is written about TB disclosure, there is a vast amount written on HIV disclosure, particularly in African contexts, where, early in the epidemic, many researchers and public health practitioners observed that people did not disclose their HIV diagnoses publicly. In these early years, this lack of public dis-closure, or talk, about HIV was viewed as an obstacle to HIV prevention. It was attributed to stigma and denial of HIV, and public health efforts tended to hinge on confessional technologies (Nguyen 2005), getting people to speak publicly about their HIV infection to break the silence. Disclosure was taken as a public health measure to combat stigma and denial and, thus, served in and of itself as a form of prevention and therapy.[1] Such an understanding has been strongly cri-tiqued by anthropologists working in Africa. For example, Deborah Durham and Frederick Klaits (2002) have shown that public concealment of HIV in Botswana was often an effort to retain mutuality and civility under difficult circumstances. In Malawi, Pauline Peters, Peter Walker, and Daimon Kambewa suggested that silence was an effort to strive for normality and thereby "control the abnormal circumstances of the rising toll of HIV-related illness and death" (2008, 662).

Despite growing ambivalence among researchers about the inherent good of disclosure, HIV disclosure persists as both an international aid technique and scholarly research focus, with an increasing emphasis on disclosures to children.[2] One dominant belief among practitioners is that parental and guardian disclo-sure of HIV to children might help children by making adult-child communi-cation easier and enabling adults and children to better prepare for the future. In such discussions, silence is viewed as something that forestalls communica-tion and relationship building and, therefore, must be broken. Take as just one of many examples an article on disclosure to children in Uganda. The authors argue: "in an era of AIDS, cultural silence about death is . . . closely linked with denial; in fact, it may be described as a *passive* form of denial, a 'hiding behind' culture, a denial of responsibility. Adults' silence towards children about death and loss may be 'excused' by saying that 'in our culture we don't talk to children about death.' This is expedient because it is easier to remain silent" (Daniel et al. 2007, 111). While the authors acknowledge that parents do not set out to harm children, they concluded that cultural silence might undermine interventions to promote children's resilience and facilitate emotional bonds between adults and children (118). Here, silence becomes equated with inaction and a failure of speech as well as with denial, not just of HIV, sex, or death, but also of parental responsibility. While aimed at increasing the resilience of children, discussions on adult disclosure to children can take on a moralizing tone, criticizing adults for not telling their children about HIV.

Tracing the ways in which children and adults were communicating about TB, I suggest, provides a critical entry point into the issue of disease disclosure, which permeates health research and programs around the world. I build on anthropological insights on concealment and silence, and pull together many forms of evidence to develop a new approach to the study of disease disclosure with children.[3] In the first sections, I focus on adult understandings of the changing burden of TB disease in their communities and their views on the risks involved in disclosing TB to their children. These sections serve as a counterpoint to public health accounts of disclosure to children that are critical of adults who do not tell their children about their disease diagnoses and that view disclosure as a quick fix to improve children's lives.

Disclosure in general, and disclosure to children in particular, is often conceptualized as a one-sided process, with one person disclosing and the other being disclosed to. Children's roles in such processes are often minimized or erased entirely. The second half and crux of this chapter is about children's experiences with naming TB and HIV. I offer an ethnography of children's silences to emphasize that silence is not the limit of adult-child communication about disease. Following the work of Carol Kidron (2009), I attend to the silent presences of TB in caring and mundane practices, material objects, and children's sentiment management.[4] Because the intertwined notions of silence and disclosure are part of discussions on many health conditions, the insights that the children offered on these topics extend well beyond studies of HIV, TB, childhood, or the southern African contexts.

THE HISTORICAL MEMORY OF TB

Since the 1980s, Zambians have witnessed dramatic political and economic changes. These changes coincided with the HIV epidemic and greatly exacerbated its effects on population health and people's abilities to manage illness in their families. In the introduction to this book, I described the spike in TB illnesses and deaths in Zambia in the 1980s and 1990s, and the continued high incidence of TB today. Though the burden of TB has substantially increased, TB was a familiar disease to Zambians even before the 1980s. TB incidence remained consistently around 100 active TB cases per every 100,000 people prior to the HIV epidemic (Mwaba 2003). This incidence only sounds low when compared to its exponential rise to more than 500 in every 100,000 people in the year 2000 and current rates that hover around 400 in 100,000 people per year.

The reality that TB has a long history in Zambia is embedded in local commentaries about TB and the mechanisms needed to control the disease.

Zambians think deeply about the causes of TB and their roles in managing the disease and preventing its effects, including its effects on children. As Julie Livingston (2005) has suggested, an analysis of people's understanding of historical change is fundamental to understanding how people think about and approach health transitions. In the context of the changing TB burden in Zambia, it is key to comprehending the ways in which adults were constructing children's risks and also how they communicate about the disease with children. I have drawn on many sources to inform this sketch of the historical memory of TB, including my research in George, conversations I had as a member of the Zambia and South African Tuberculosis and AIDS Reduction study (ZAMSTAR) team in other areas of Lusaka, the Copperbelt, Central Province, and Southern Province, and also my analysis of transcripts of interviews and group discussions carried out by the ZAMSTAR study team.[5]

When older Zambians talked about TB in the past, they often invoked, perhaps not an ideal past but a past in which TB contagion was under control. Take for example an elderly traditional healer who talked about how people grappled with the burden of TB in her community. She described the changes: "People are now concerned with the origins of TB and how they are going to go about managing the disease because too many people are dying. If we think back to how we used to live and life now, things are really different. A long time ago, when a person is suffering from TB, medicines used to be sought until the patient was completely cured. We used to care."[6] She described how the way people live now has decreased care for the sick, making the claim that "we used to care," a "we" that seems to refer broadly to health systems, healers, communities, and families. People made strong connections between the economic and political shifts in the country, the inability to control the disease, and a declining moral order. A woman in her sixties illustrated these connections in her assessment of the rise in TB. She said:

> TB was there in the past but it used to be curable because it was well managed. Even at the hospitals in the past, TB patients used to be isolated. But now it's not managed well, patients are careless; they even share their food with children and end up infecting everybody. In the past when a person was found with TB, the entire household would also go for TB tests and if there were others found with TB, they would all be put on treatment. But now it's not the same, if one is found with TB, they are simply told to go back home. The entire household ends up contracting the disease. Even the doctors are not enough; it is each man for himself.[7]

The differences between life now and life back then, people explained, were vast. Older residents recalled early TB control measures, including social control measures, positively as they made sense of the rise in TB. They suggested that hospitals and clinics used to have good control measures and that biomedical and traditional medicines were able to cure TB. Families had the things they needed to care for TB patients and the ability to put systems in place to prevent TB's spread because food was more plentiful and houses were not as overcrowded. Patients adhered to social norms that prevented the spread of TB and "followed the rules" of treatment when they were sick.[8]

The moral order in today's Zambia was at the heart of many of the comments on TB. When people talked about the breakdown in the moral order that prevented infection in the past, they did not accuse members of all social categories equally. Most frequently, they implicated women and youth in the rise in TB. As one man suggested in conversation about the changes that have prompted the rise in TB today: "Nowadays children discipline their parents instead of the other way round.[9] The human rights are a problem because when you try to discipline the child if the child is drinking and engaging in bad behavior, the child may take you to the police for child abuse. So now the children are free to do anything they want. That's why they are catching TB."[10] In this quote, he was referring to the global discourses and programs he believes have subverted the power of older generations to control younger people.

Women, too, were seen as not following traditions as they once had. Traditions included an array of practices that differed by locale but almost always hinged on women's abilities to contaminate others at critical times, such as when they were menstruating or after a miscarriage or abortion. During these times, women were supposed to observe certain rules such as not cooking or having sex to avoid contamination. As one older man explained in a group discussion about the changing spread of TB: "At that time [in the past], if a woman aborted, she would stay for some time without sleeping with a man. But nowadays you meet these women in bars because of poverty and so [they are] spreading TB. They do not even consider using condoms."[11] He combined older notions of contamination with more recent interpretations of HIV as preventable through condom use, while also conflating TB and HIV. His comments showed how women were receiving blame for the spread of the disease, even when the structural inequalities that women faced were acknowledged.

People classified TB to demarcate differences in the past and present, as well as differentially assign blame. Take for example the classifications of "new TB" and "TB of the past." Both new TB and TB of the past exist in present-day Zambia, but they carry very different meanings for TB sufferers, families, and onlookers (Bond and Nyblade 2006). New TB has been associated with HIV; it is hard to cure and more deadly, and it carries the weight of the moral transgressions associated with HIV. People understood TB of the past as transmissible, but it was considered treatable and less shameful, primarily because it was disentangled from HIV and AIDS.

People diagnosed with TB worked to make sense of their suffering through categories such as new TB and TB of the past. Kelvyn Kabaso, a father of several young children, struggled to understand why he had TB. While he never invoked HIV, and I am uncertain of his HIV status, he expressed to me on a number of occasions that his diagnosis was a source of shame for his children and worry for him. His family did not have a history of TB from which he could draw to account for his illness. He repeatedly said, "Jean, I am the first person in my family to suffer from this disease," insinuating that he had brought the disease into the family, making it something other than TB of the past or "family TB." Instead, it was a disease for which he bore responsibility for catching and potentially spreading and one from which his family may never recover.

Comparisons with the past offer insight into how children and TB patients were seen within the current TB epidemic in Zambia. Take for example the woman I quoted earlier who identified that "patients are careless; they even share their food with children." Many adults I spoke with punctuated their descriptions of the adult actions that caused the rise in TB incidence with references to the dangers adult TB patients presented to children. Their statements revealed blame and also their vulnerabilities. The reality that even children become sick with the TB of today drove this point home.

Children at Risk and Adults to Blame

The peak age range of people diagnosed with active TB in Zambia has been estimated at twenty to thirty-five years old.[12] In clinics it was rare to see very young TB sufferers on treatment.[13] Children have long been left out of public health and medical protocols for managing TB because of the lower burden of TB in children, the difficulties in diagnosing children's TB, and the dominant public health belief that children's TB is less infectious and, thus, less of a public health emergency.[14] Children may not be the primary targets of many TB interventions. However, their risk of TB is the subject of intense concern among residents of George and other heavily TB-affected urban and peri-urban areas in Zambia.

Unpublished interviews and group discussions carried out within the ZAMSTAR study give weight to just how concerned some Zambians were about exposing children to TB or having a friend or relative expose them to the disease. Researchers asked forty-six men and women who had TB to describe who in their communities was most at risk of getting TB. Twenty-nine out of forty-six respondents (63 percent) named children as most at risk, at risk, or in need of protection from becoming infected with TB.

We might envision their concerns about children, in part, as an "early warning system" (Biehl and Petryna 2013a, 18), in which people have identified a real health concern for children and their families.[15] Take for example a conversation

I had with a longtime resident of George who volunteered at George Health Centre. He told me about how tricky it was for anyone to identify TB-related coughs. Speaking hypothetically, he said: "You don't know that I have TB, but I'll start coughing. And I may say that it's an ordinary cough when it is TB, and then I'll take him [pointing to a child nearby] and other children." TB exposure in George is real, and no one can avoid it. Total avoidance of TB would translate as social isolation and a lapse in sociality. Residents of George discussed a number of places where they might be exposed to TB. People viewed taverns as a primary site of TB transmission. These were implicated because of their association with smoking, drinking, and promiscuous sex. However, people also recognized that TB might be spread at funerals and during the visitation and care of the sick. In the views of many commentators, the spaces of a funeral house[16] and the hospital, clinic, or home where a sick person rests were decidedly different from taverns because, while taverns represented moral transgressions, attending funerals and visiting the sick were moral obligations. Not attending a funeral or not visiting an ill person demonstrated an extreme lapse in sociality. Such a lapse in sociality lends itself to gossip about the quality of the heart and motivations of a person. In the act of going (or not going) to a funeral house or the home of a sick person, social ties are built and broken. Residents developed strategies to minimize their exposure, such as sitting near windows or doors. However, they also realized that exposure was a fact of everyday life.

When Zambians emphasized children's risks of TB, they were conveying ideas about children's inabilities to protect themselves within such a setting. Many people expressed to me a view that children were unaware of TB and protective measures. They connected children's susceptibility to TB to their level of social, emotional, and intellectual maturity. For example, when I asked a volunteer TB treatment supporter at George Health Centre if children should be told about TB disease in their households, he replied: "If they are under ten, even if you tell [them], they won't understand what is TB, what is HIV.[17] They are blank." Residents suggested that children's lack of understanding and their "childish" actions put them at risk of contracting the disease. For example, I was told: "children like to play in the dirt and so they can easily get TB." Playing in the dirt is a marker of childhood. Children fashion dolls and animals out of mud and play games with their friends on the ground. Adults connected children's play with TB sufferers who "spit anyhow," and spitting made playing in the dirt dangerous.

In addition to playing in the dirt, children climbed on those who suffered from TB, and they hugged and kissed them to show affection. Such acts encouraged the sick in Zambia, where love was viewed as integral to recovery. But children's proximity also became a source of concern because it increased a child's exposure to TB. Adults worried that children would eat TB patients' leftover food, a real concern in a setting where children rely on scavenged and leftover foods to meet their nutritional needs. The foods given to TB patients tempted children because they were luxuries not eaten on a daily basis, such as fruits, meats, eggs, and juices.

Adults constructed themselves as actors and children as victims within the epidemic. "Careless" adults were blamed for giving TB to children. Children were at risk of getting TB "because they can get it from an adult who has TB."[18] With children's innocence as a persistent theme in commentaries about TB, the guilt and responsibility of adults who did not protect children from TB was highlighted. Such a construction has placed high demands on adults—particularly women—to forestall the spread of the disease and protect children.

The presumption of guilt and the great responsibility to protect children was particularly worrisome for TB sufferers I knew. As one woman suffering from TB pointed out, "it is not good to spread the disease to children." She and others worried not just about social blame, but about the very real suffering that TB might cause the child and the strain it would place on household resources. Sick adults were put in a difficult position in which they had to ensure that TB was not spread to children and yet they had few resources at hand to do so. These evaluations and material challenges shaped how they chose to reveal or conceal their disease.

Adults: Revealing and Concealing

The evaluations within popular histories and taxonomies of TB placed adults in precarious positions as they navigated a complex moral terrain where they were alternately feared, stigmatized, viewed as careless, and called upon to act responsibly. TB sufferers and other adult caregivers expressed a sense of urgency to ensure children's safety. This urgency included managing children's fears and providing them with material and emotional supports, and these included managing children's knowledge of TB. It was, in fact, often impossible for me to disentangle social constructions of TB disease and TB spread from ideas about disclosure to children. Take for example the connection one woman made between concealing knowledge of TB from children and protecting them from disease: "If the children are fifteen years and above, I can tell them that I have TB. If the children are young, I can make sure I prevent them from getting TB." Her linking of TB disclosure to age makes two ideas evident: protection is tied to knowledge and younger children need protection rather than knowledge.

In the introduction to this chapter, I described my conversations with Mr. Simwonde and other guardians who did not wish to mention TB to the children in their households. Instead of seeing disclosure as protective, they identified concealment as a form of protection and spoke of the illness through other terms. Some described it as malaria. Others called it *matenda*, a Nyanja word that translates as sickness or disease. Still other families referred to illness as *mendo*, or legs, a term used during a sickness when a person's legs become weak or they can no longer walk.

An exception to this concealment was when a guardian could completely divorce their TB from HIV, which became especially clear in one mother's explanation for how and why she told her daughters Abby and Chiko about her TB. The mother, Elesia, knew that people were skeptical of statements that deny HIV when you have TB. So as proof that she did not have HIV, Elesia invoked her family history of TB, referring to her disease as "family TB" and "TB of the past." She also wore a yellow wristband as additional proof. The wristband was one of many given out after a person received an HIV test from a New Start HIV Counseling and Testing Centre. New Start Centres are directly managed or franchised by Population Services International (PSI), a nongovernmental organization that is based in Washington, DC, and works in Zambia and other countries. Written on the wristbands was the question: "I know, Do you?" Wristbands were given to everyone who received a test, regardless of the result. They served as a form of branded advertising meant to, in the words used to describe the intervention on PSI's website, "help create awareness and generate demand for HIV Counseling and Testing."

The wristbands are a means of public disclosure—disclosure that one has tested for HIV. Elesia had never been to a New Start Centre and had borrowed the yellow wristband from a friend. She told me that people in George know that you do not have HIV when you wear the wristband. This was, of course, not the type of message the developers of the campaign had in mind. Nevertheless, the wristband was a highly visible cue indicating that Elesia did not have HIV. It, along with other cues, freed Elesia to speak of her TB diagnosis with her daughters. When I asked if they knew about her TB, she said: "I told them 'Do not worry, I will recover because it is not AIDS.'" Elesia's actions and statements suggest that HIV, rather than TB, is a primary, underlying concern when considering TB disclosure. She also demonstrated the lengths to which a person must go to prove HIV seronegativity when HIV is the default expectation.

With the exception of Elesia, most guardians in my study did not name TB when talking to the children in their households or extended families. They gave two main reasons, each of which carried a number of implied concerns, including the link between HIV and TB and the association of TB with moral transgressions, suffering, and death. They worried that children might reveal information about TB in inappropriate ways. Encapsulated in this concern was the idea that children may use the term TB haphazardly or disclose a family's private information at school or in their neighborhood.

The idea that children do not keep information private shaped the advice patients and families received from clinic workers and volunteers at George

Health Centre, where most people in George received TB treatment. Explaining why they advised people not to tell their young children, one longtime worker told me that, if children are told, "They'll be saying, 'Eh, my relative is suffering from TB.' You know children, they don't hide." Children's explicit naming of TB was viewed as potentially harmful to the TB patient, the child, and the family. The reasons why people did not want other people to know or openly verbalize TB were frequently related to issues of care. Explicit naming of TB was seen as harmful to a sick person's well-being because of TB's association with death. Adult caregivers worried that a child may reference TB in ways that might cause the patient to give up or make them think about their prognosis. They also worried that children would sever their own relationships unknowingly by sharing news of a guardian's diagnosis. For example, Mr. Simwonde explained: "If I told him, he could have explained the news [to others, especially to his friends]. He can simply be disappointed from his friend. From his side, he cannot feel right."

The second reason that adults gave for not telling children was the belief that disease knowledge had an effect on a child's well-being. They worried that their children might reject them or be disappointed in them. They suggested that a guardian's TB or HIV status could prompt children to think too much [*kuganiza maningi*] and, when people start to "think too much," they might easily lose hope and feel isolated. In this view, knowledge has an effect on people, and specific knowledge has a negative effect on children. When I asked Mr. Simwonde to explain the process of thinking too much as it relates to disclosure of TB to his son, he told me in English: "He is too young. He can have [an] inferior complex—this brings life expectancy of a human to be little. It cannot build confidence [in him]." Mr. Simwonde's statement attests to the ways in which illness can reduce a person to mere existence. However, it is not the person who is sick that he refers to. He recounts, instead, the ways in which parental illness can reduce a child's life.

Unlike in much of the HIV disclosure literature, stigma and denial were not the main analytical categories that drove nondisclosure in my study. Instead, what drove nondisclosure was a guardian's effort to retain relationships and normative roles and identities under highly uncertain conditions. Rather than constituting bad parenting, not telling was an effort to be a good parent.

Children: Knowing and Performing

I was faced with a dilemma when I began working with the children. I wanted to respect adults' views of protection and risk, but I also did not wish to mislead the children. I decided to approach the situation by not bringing up any disease names during the study unless the children spoke them first. While this approach was much more in line with local modes of talk about sickness that I described above, in which disease names were de-emphasized or circumvented in place of other expressions, it yielded little information about TB specifically. Several months after I began the research, I had yet to hear any of the children use the terms TB or HIV in my presence or the guardians use those terms in conversation when their children were present. Whenever I asked the children what their family members were suffering from, they told me "legs," "malaria," or just "disease." Even Abby, Elesia's daughter, did not speak out loud about TB.

About five months after I met many of the children, I asked them to participate in what we called "children's workshops," as a way to for me to gather different insights on children's disease knowledge and experiences of household illness. The children's workshops took place in a freestanding building, known as the Demonstration Room, which sat on the grounds of George Health Centre. The children came for the children's workshops in groups of approximately ten children during three separate afternoons. We played games and had group discussions, and the children created role plays.

The novelty of the children's workshops was the purposeful exclusion of adults, an aspect that thrilled the children and met with approval from adults, if not a little teasing about when they should come for an adults' workshop. The theory behind the workshops was that knowledge is always situated. That is, the settings of research and the people present shape the ways in which children act and respond to research questions (Edwards and Alldred 1999). Group discussions offer a valuable addition to household ethnography because questions can be framed in more general terms (Morgan et al. 2002), whereas questions about illness in the presence of a sick family member might always feel personalized, even when phrased in general terms.

During the children's workshops, I provided a rough framework of activities that focused on illness generally, rather than TB or HIV specifically. I wanted the sessions to be guided by children's illness concerns and not by biomedical categories and labels that may or may not hold relevance to their daily lives. And because I was gathering a range of children who did not previously know one another, I wanted the research to be sensitive to each individual child's suffering and circumstances. Twelve-year-old Musa, for example, had watched his older brother die two months before the workshop. Ten-year-old Sarafina's mother was again bedridden, her condition worsening. Ten-year-old Rhoda's "small mother," her mother's sister, was also bedridden. And the sheer number of TB sufferers in eight-year-old Gift's household—his grandmother, grandfather, sister, and uncle—infused daily life with uncertainty.

"Living in a House with a Sick Person"

Musa, Sarafina, Rhoda, and Gift formed one of ten groups across three workshops that acted out a role play on the theme: "living in a house with a sick person." The theme was the only direction I gave the children, and I avoided terms such as care, so as not to influence the direction of the role plays. I had yet to hear any of the children use the terms TB or HIV. During the months prior to the workshop, Musa had told me that his brother was suffering from *mendo* [legs]. Sarafina said that her mother had malaria, and Gift and Rhoda talked about their family members' illnesses as *matenda* [sickness].

In the role play I am about to describe, Musa played the doctor, Gift played a sick man, and Rhoda and Sarafina played Gift's aunt and mother. The group started with the sick man arriving at a clinic with his mother and aunt. The doctor examined the sick man, exclaiming: "He! He's caught TB. I am going to give you this medicine. The way you're supposed to take this medicine. At night, you drink two. And again in the morning at 6, you take two. And again, in the daytime, you take two after eating. Do you understand?" The doctor then handed an imaginary bag of pills to the sick man's aunt, saying: "If it doesn't work, you come back." The three children playing the sick man, mother, and aunt walked slowly to the other side of the Demonstration Room, representing a long distance between clinic and home. Once home, the sick man lay on a bench, with his mother and aunt watching over him. The mother and aunt gave the man medicine, watched him, fed him, told him to sleep, and woke him up to take more medicine. After a couple of quiet moments passed, the aunt decided: "The medicine is too big and it is not working."

The family set out for the clinic and, when they arrived, the doctor told the man: "It seems like your TB is too strong." He then reexamined him, patting his arm and talking in a low voice. He listened to the man's lungs and offered a new diagnosis: "*Imwe, muli na double* [You, you've got double]." To clarify his euphemism, he repeated the diagnosis: "*Muli na* HIV *na* TB [you have HIV and TB]." With this news, the doctor explained that the man needed further medicine and injections. After giving him an injection, the family returned to their fictive home across the Demonstration Room, never mentioning the words HIV or TB. They altered their daily routines to remind the man to take his medicine. They encouraged him to sleep and eat. And they spent long intervals silently watching over him. Eleven minutes after the role play began, the children ended it. The man's illness had yet to be cured and he remained sick, lying on the bench until the audience applauded.

Across the ten role plays conducted by different children during three separate workshops, all but one role play focused on detailed accounts of TB treatment. Even Mulenga, Mr. Simwonde's son, played a doctor treating a patient who had a combination of what he diagnosed as "TB and sugar disease." Their TB diagnoses were not, however, definitive diagnoses. In each role play, the sicknesses seemed to get worse and involve numerous trips to the clinic. New diagnoses and treatments layered onto old ones, and there remained much uncertainty about diagnosis, treatment, and prognosis.

Presence in Advice and Isolation

During the children's workshops, I asked the children to develop lists of the sicknesses that most concerned them. On their lists, the children included a range of biomedical and local terms for diseases, as well as certain things that observers might not consider to be diseases, such as ARVs.[19] They listed TB in all three workshops. After they developed the list, Olivious went through each item, asking a similar set of questions about each. When she reached TB, the children were quiet. In one group, she finally asked: "Have any of you talked about TB with your family?" To this question, one girl said: "My grandfather, mother, and my sister suffered from TB and took medication." The phrasing of the girl's answer prompted Olivious to also rephrase her question: "How do you know when someone has TB?" This was a question on which the children had much to say.

Children pointed to learning about TB from adults through restrictions and changes in the household that were intended to avoid transmission. Agnes replied: "I was told by my grandmother when they came back from the clinic, 'your elder sister is suffering from TB, so you should not use the same cups and plates with her.'" As an aside, the adults in Agnes's household emphasized several times that they did not disclose Rebecca's disease label until well into her treatment, and only in response to Agnes's persistent questioning about the medicines that Rebecca was taking. Elesia's daughter, Abby, replied to our question: "When my mother came back from the clinic she was using her own utensils and we were told not to eat left out food by her or use her face towel." Several girls spoke of not being able to sleep in the same bed as mothers or aunts, an aspect that was so upsetting to Abby's sister, Chiko, that, when using my tape recorder, she suggested that she and Abby should also get sick. This way, she reasoned, they could again sleep with their mother.

Children associate diagnoses with their own and the sick person's sanctioned and unsanctioned behavior. Only a few years prior to my study, the standard clinical advice given to people who suffered from TB was isolation. To avoid transmission, TB patients and their families were told to eat and sleep separately. During my research, nurses and TB treatment supporters—volunteers who assisted at the health center and provided community outreach—often talked about this advice as outdated and stigmatizing.[20] Once on treatment for two or more weeks, TB sufferers are usually not considered to be infectious, and much more transmission occurs prior to diagnosis. For this reason, health practitioners stressed the importance of not abandoning those who suffer from TB. When I asked a volunteer who gave support to people who were on TB treatment about the advice he gave when someone first received their diagnosis, he told me:

First on the eating system: You see, many people are dying with TB because after being diagnosed with the TB, they were being isolated. That was depressing other people's minds [the minds of those with TB] so they die of depression. This was not good. So we introduced using separate plates for relish. If it's rice, then each one has his separate plate. In the environment, especially where that person sleeps should be very clean. In the morning he should bathe. The windows should be opened. Children should be isolated in the other room alone.

The items he listed corresponded with the range of changes that children noted in their discussions of how they knew someone had TB. However, despite his overt focus on how to remain close without transmitting TB, his statement demonstrates the continued concern over children's proximity to TB sufferers. Children received both messages—about avoidance and also about remaining close as good care.

Presence in Children's Caregiving

During the household research, I asked each child to make drawings of "taking care of a sick person." These drawings were designed as a way for children to illustrate their ideas about care and a tool for me to use to engage them in conversation about caregiving. Ten-year-old Annie's drawing offers one such example. Annie lived in a one-room rental unit with her mother, Enelesi, and her "sister," the daughter of Annie's oldest sister, who was deceased. In Annie's drawing of "taking care of a sick person," she showed just how sick Enelesi had become and many aspects of how she viewed her role in giving care. Though Enelesi was adamant that she had not disclosed her TB or HIV diagnoses to Annie, the presence of TB was clear in her drawing, as it was in the other children's drawings.

Annie depicted a set of four scenes on a white sheet of paper. At the top, she showed her mom waiting in bed. In her words, "She wants to vomit so I hold her hand to take her outside." In the middle, she depicted herself giving her mother her daily medicine with a glass of drinking water. Next to that scene, she drew herself "chatting and eating" with her mother. Annie showed how she and her mother used clinical advice of eating with separate bowls to continue to have their meals together, making tangible and reinforcing their connection to each other.[21] Other children showed themselves involved in bringing special foods to their sick guardians, particularly fruits, which are luxury items in George and a symbol of love when given to the sick. The final picture on the page was Annie accompanying her mother to George Health Centre to collect medicine, something that Annie did not in fact do, but these visits were a part of her mother's weekly routine to collect TB medications and ARVs. TB and HIV are present in all four drawings. Even though Annie's mother did not wish to tell Annie about

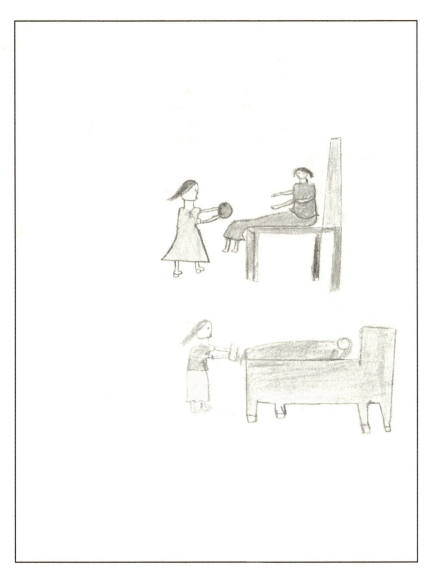

Fig. 3.1 Drawing of Irene taking care of a sick person. She gives the sick person an orange and drinking water. Drawing by Irene, age twelve.

her TB or HIV diagnoses, Annie was involved in her mother's care, a process that gave her a detailed knowledge of the diseases.

Special foods and medicines were integral actors in child-guardian interactions (see fig. 3.1). They gave children and adults a way to address illness and suffering as well as nurture each other without directly naming a disease. Take, for example, a story that eleven-year-old Rose recorded in February 2008, seven months after her grandmother had begun TB treatment. I had given her a series of pictures to view as she told stories on my tape recorder. To tell her stories, she hid in an empty room in her family's home, a common tactic children employed when using the recorders. The children rarely wanted family members to listen to what they had to say. Speaking on a picture of a person lying in bed, surrounded by family members, Rose said:

> This is my father. He is suffering from TB, and he is telling his children: "I am sick my children. But my children, I am taking my medicine. I went to the hospital and I was given this medicine. In case I might forget my dosage, you should remind me. And they have also given the vitamins. These are the TB tablets. I was also told to eat a lot of food and fruits." He later got better because he followed his medication very well. My father didn't die. I love you, Dad.

In Rose's story, her fictive father does not name TB so much as make evident his bodily needs, manage their fears, and give them caregiving roles. There is a subtle but important distinction between this form of making a disease known and the more Euro-American assumption about disclosing as the act of revealing a name to a sickness or condition. His making known—or disclosure—was about caring actions that occurred between people. It was about relationships and responsibilities to one another, rather than indicative of the ends of them. In Rose's words, "My father didn't die."

Concealment as Emotion Work

Returning to the children's role plays on living with a sick person, a consistent theme across the role plays was the explicit naming of TB by the children who played the doctors but no other children in the groups. The role plays seemed to make a clear point: just as adults avoid saying TB, children also engage in tactical avoidances and concealments. In their strategic usage and avoidance of naming TB in their role plays, as well as in their daily encounters in their homes, children demonstrated an understanding that naming disease has effects on others and on their relationships, something that is hardly different from my observations about how adults approached naming with children.

I have documented only one case in which two girls named TB and HIV in front of their sick uncle. Mateo, their uncle, had moved to their house from nearby when he could no longer care for himself. After he moved in, the children reportedly used the words TB and HIV directly in front of their uncle, saying both diagnoses loudly when talking with neighbors and friends about Mateo. Family members viewed their direct naming to and near Mateo as a rupture in care for the sick man. During several of my visits, Mateo's brother, the head of the household and father of one girl and an uncle of the other, worried aloud to me. He believed that their direct naming might have harmful effects on Mateo, caus-ing him to "think too much" about his own future and lose hope for recovery. And even though the girls carried out much of the work of caring for the man, such as bringing him food and preparing his bathwater, their work was never acknowledged as "care." When I asked Mateo and other household members if they might consider the girls' activities as care, they spoke instead of the girls' naming, avoidances, and the negative sentiments they expressed when giving him food, preparing his bathwater, and performing other chores for him. Recall earlier in the chapter that this was the type of behavior that adults feared might happen.

The children could not have been aware of Mateo's HIV seropositivity because even he did not know at the time. His HIV tests were negative. Only a test at the very end of my study showed that he was, in fact, positive. I cannot be sure why the children disliked their uncle so much or of the history of their relationship with him. What I do know is this: since his arrival, the burden of care for him had been placed on them and caring for him subsumed household resources and took the girls away from their studies and other activities.

In all but this one household, not naming, revealing, or confirming seemed to serve as a critical part of children's attempts to give care to parents and guardians. Rather than something that prevented care and relationship building, conceal-ment served as a mode of care and an effort to negotiate belonging at a time when their proximity to the sick person and the household was in threat. We might consider concealment, then, as just one aspect of children's range of prac-tices to nurture the sick, such as reminding guardians to take their medicine, making food and preparing bathwater, cleaning the house, attending school without complaint, or—in two brothers' case—lying to their mother about going to school when they were out making money to support the household. It was important to many children to sit with the sick, make them laugh, and encourage them that they would get better. This demonstrates the children's keen aware-ness of the need to manage emotions, what anthropologist Arlie Hochschild has called "emotion work" (Hochschild 2003). We should not underestimate the importance of children's emotion work in households dealing with illness or the amount of effort children put into managing their own and others emotions.

Children's emotion work related to their worries that relatives might give up, a process that could lead to death. In one of eleven-year-old Paul Kangwa's recordings, for example, he made clear how pain and suffering from TB might diminish a person's desire to live, inducing them to give up on life. Speaking in the voice of a sick father, Paul said: "Let me die. It's okay even if I die." In the recorded conversation Paul enacted, he worked to persuade his father that he would get better. By following the rules around talk about particular diseases, children showed themselves to be responsive to the needs of relatives. There were significant rewards for such behavior. It ensured their continued presence in households and proximity to relatives; it helped them cultivate and reaffirm their relationships with their relatives; and it helped them stay alive.

Seeing children's concealments as emotion work demands that we recognize the lengths to which children may go to nurture the sick. While much of children's emotion work went unnoticed by adults in George, as it does in many places in the world, Annie's mother, Enelesi, described the value of Annie's efforts. Recall Annie's four scenes of caring for her mother. During the time Annie was drawing those scenes, Enelesi and I spoke about her illness and Annie's care. She said to me as she glanced over at Annie: "When your heart is heavy with something, there is always someone who will control you. When there are children, they will tell you that it's all right and the sun will rise tomorrow." Children, Enelesi explained, helped manage the negative sentiments held by others, which might harm her or inhibit her recovery from TB and her management of HIV. Enelesi's statement highlights a particular aspect of the TB and HIV epidemics that I have not yet discussed, which is that Zambians sometimes attributed their afflictions in part to invisible or supernatural forces, such as witchcraft or Satanism, caused by a lover, neighbor, friend, or family member.[22] My point is that children's emotion work can have a range of interpretations and effects on the ill, which deserve acknowledgment.

When TB Is Named

I return now to Elesia, the mother of two girls—Abby and Chiko—who told her daughters immediately and directly about her TB diagnosis. They represent the only case in my study where a caregiver explicitly named TB. Their situation offers an alternative view that may serve as a challenge to Euro-American assumptions that naming disease has beneficial effects on both children and the sick. As I mentioned in the introduction to this book, Elesia's sister, brother, uncle, and other relatives gathered together just after Elesia's TB diagnosis to discuss who would take care of Elesia and the children. Elesia had been sick for a long time, but it was her TB diagnosis that prompted the family to separate Elesia from her children. The plan was contested by Elesia and her children, but eventually put into place when the family moved Elesia to her sister's house in another low-income settlement on the opposite side of the city. The girls moved in with their uncle (see chapter 2).

Several weeks after the separation, Olivious and I visited Abby and Chiko at their uncle's house. Tired of drawing, the girls asked for my tape recorder and started shyly singing into it. Once they tired of singing, Olivious suggested that they might take the recorder in the bedroom and *bisa* [hide] from us. That way, she explained, they could play more freely with the recorder. When they returned from the bedroom, they asked us to play back the following recorded conversation:

ABBY: Us here, we want our mother to come back and start living with her because we are used to staying with our mother. Chiko, come and say something.

CHIKO: My mother should get better.

ABBY: My mother should get better, I am praying for her so that we start living together, it's just her who is only getting sick.

CHIKO: We should also get sick.

ABBY: Why can't she just get better, she is just getting sick alone and being ordered around by other people. Me, I want my mother to get better so that we can start living together. I miss my mother a lot. I just want her to get better and come home. We are fed up of always going to visit her there. We want her to come home. We are used to staying with her and not other people.

CHIKO: What I dreamt today, I dreamt that people from the clinic had come to tell me that my mother has died.

Olivious and I were the people from the clinic. My heart sank after hearing that line, and I phoned Elesia immediately so that she and the girls could talk. The girls told her about Chiko's dream. She reassured them that she was taking her medicine and already feeling much better.

Abby and Chiko's situation was interesting because, at first glance and from a public health angle, they seemed to have several advantages over the other children. Their mother told them immediately that she had TB. The family put a plan in place for their care, and their maternal aunt took care of Elesia during the initial stages of her TB treatment when Elesia's care was very time consuming and her TB was possibly still infectious. Still, the situation looked quite different from Abby and Chiko's points of view. Even though they knew Elesia's clinical diagnosis, their inability to observe their mother's illness trajectory increased their concerns about their mother's recovery and their own future. The children expressed that they derived important benefits from being in close proximity to their mothers, namely the ability to ensure that she received care. In Abby's view, proximity rather than disclosure was the foremost indicator of good care for both her and her mother.

Conclusion

In activist, public health, and media reports, HIV disclosure has been viewed as a child's right, something that promotes an individual child's resilience and strengthens communication between adults and children and moves children to action. The problem in such discussions is not the virus per se but how illness and death affect children materially and emotionally. The solution is to focus on a particular type of communication that is assumed to prompt even further communication, which will then allay the negative effects of AIDS-related diseases and deaths on children as well as adults. This solution misses the mark in part because of its "immodest claims of causality" (Farmer 1999): that naming is helpful and not naming can cause more harm. Naming HIV (or not) figures as both the problem and the answer to adult-child communication, relationship building, and well-being. Such a view elides the pressing economic and political factors that shape how all people—young and old—communicate about suffering. As this chapter has shown, focusing only on naming attends to just one small aspect of communication strategies and ignores other forms of knowing and communicating.

The issue of disclosure is one that will remain at the center of debates on children's protection, provision, and participation in the context of the HIV epidemic. I suspect it will also become a prominent issue in TB programming because of the recent global attention to tuberculosis in children. To an extent, it has also been identified as an important topic in the study of cancer and other diseases in the United States and around the world. For this reason, I would like to conclude this chapter with three points that my study raises for future research on disclosure.

First, by calling attention to children's detailed knowledge and tactical use of disease names such as TB or HIV, I do not intend to suggest that the children were completely certain about the biomedical diagnoses of their relatives. I do believe that uncertainty and confusion around diagnosis and prognosis were part of the children's experiences, as the children vividly showed in their role plays. But uncertainty and confusion were also part of the experience for the TB sufferers themselves, other adult family members, health workers in George, and even me. People expressed uncertainties when a person became sicker when taking TB medicine and/or ARVs. They expressed confusion when HIV tests revealed contradictory results through time, or when TB could be found only in an X-ray and not in a sputum smear. And, while most people in George struggled with poor health during treatment, there were a few who recovered their health in miraculous ways. To borrow Abby's words: "They come back even better than they were before." This too raised questions about the validity of diagnosis and prognosis. Perhaps the research and discussion on disclosure has focused too much on certainties in a way that erases the lived experience of uncertainty within illness, particularly in resource-poor areas. For in most studies and reports on disclosure, disclosure is framed as a yes or no variable. As a yes or no variable, we cannot understand how uncertainties shape the ways people know and talk about disease.

Second, and not unrelated, despite the confusion and uncertainty around TB and HIV, children living with ill adults often had nuanced understandings of TB and HIV/AIDS, as well as biomedical treatments and caregiving for both. Children's detailed knowledge of disease—expressed in the role plays and in their private tape-recordings—demonstrates the limitations of a view that considers children as unaware or focuses on naming as the only way of knowing. Disclosure is a process, rather than a discrete event on which all other knowledge and action is built. By focusing solely on naming disease, public health actors have assumed that disease knowledge is encapsulated in a name or precipitates from an event. Instead, disclosure comes in many forms and knowledge of illness processes is built through interactions.

My work calls for an extreme broadening of definitions of disclosure to include the silent presences and relationship-building practices, including the material objects used to communicate about a disease and specific forms of context-specific emotion work. As I have shown, children actively collected knowledge of diagnosis and prognosis. They gathered knowledge through attention to small signs, inscribed on their sick relatives' bodies and materially present in their homes. This suggests the importance of attending to multiple ways of communicating about disease, rather than just one. Drawings such as Annie's drawing of the four scenes of taking care of her mother raise a critical point. The drawings show the fallacy in assumptions that children are passive, uninvolved, and unable to communicate until they have been directly told about disease.

Finally, children make decisions on a daily basis about how and when to communicate about disease with family members, friends, neighbors, or a visiting anthropologist. They know the socially appropriate spaces to express their knowledge of TB or HIV and AIDS and where and when to remain quiet or use euphemisms and indirect references. This suggests that it is just as important to understand children's concealments as it is to understand what they do and do not know, or what they have and have not been told. Children experience and respond to a range of actions that stigmatize, blame, or shame people who are diagnosed with TB or HIV. As I have shown in both the guardian's and children's responses to naming TB, sometimes not naming, not knowing, or not confirming were the only ways in which people were able to hold each other close.

CHAPTER 4

Following the Medicine

George Health Centre is the only government-run health facility in George.[1] The clinic is set in the oldest section of the residential area, along a dusty, narrow, and deeply grooved road. It has one single-car entrance for a slow but steady stream of hired vehicles taxiing individuals too sick to walk, cars driven by the few nurses who can afford them, run-down Ministry of Health land cruisers, and expensive all-terrain vehicles belonging to internationally supported projects.[2] Most residents of George walk or are carried through this entrance. The very sick are pushed in wheelbarrows, with blankets protecting them from the morning chill and the gaze of onlookers.

Current policies on TB treatment make traversing between home and clinic a daily, weekly, and then monthly activity. TB medications are the lifeblood of the clinic's TB treatment efforts. In accordance with the World Health Organization's guidelines on TB control—directly observed treatment, short-course (DOTS)—TB medications do not flow freely from the clinic's pharmacy. Instead, a nurse doles them out on a regular basis and monitors their flow to ensure that patients do not discard, forget, or sell them over the long course of treatment. TB medicines come with many rules for patients to follow:

Take in the morning.
Drink with water.
Eat plenty of good foods.
Do not drink alcohol or smoke.
Rest.

They come with similar rules for family members:

Help the patient take their medicine.
Be patient with them.

Encourage them.

Buy them healthy food and cook for them.

Let the patient rest.

Keep the patient and their surroundings clean.

Let fresh air circulate.

Above all else, make sure that the patient takes their medicine.

Even though TB medication has been around for a long time in Zambia and elsewhere in the world, TB medicines and the many rules that accompany them are, in many respects, new in George. Their presence is a result of substantial global and national shifts in TB control during the early twenty-first century. Treatment entered George with gusto as the nation aligned its TB control effort with global mandates at this time, and substantial international funding followed. Clinicians and community members in George opened their arms to these medicines and the rules that accompanied them, after struggling to manage the effects of TB for many years without sufficient supplies of medicine or other resources. In many respects, the rules of TB treatment brought a sense of empowerment. There was finally something clinicians, family members, and TB sufferers could do about an epidemic that was killing their loved ones.

I am interested in the social implications of such substantial attention to patient adherence to medication—not just for TB, but also many diseases in which medicines serve as the primary solution to prevention, treatment, or cure. More specifically, I join other anthropologists in examining how universal treatment programs have shaped everyday efforts to direct life projects (Biehl 2005; Koch 2006, 2013). Erin Koch (2006), for example, has shown the unexpected consequence of DOTS-based programming in a prison in postsocialist Georgia. She observed that prisoners were trafficking TB-infected sputum, the bodily substance that contains TB bacilli if a person has pulmonary TB. Prisoners who did not have TB obtained and used the infected sputum of TB sufferers to achieve positive TB diagnoses on regular sputum tests given by prison authorities. Such a diagnosis (when a prisoner was not caught) allowed the prisoner access to better housing, food, and medical care while in prison. Koch characterized such subterfuge as a form of agency. Universal treatment programs, as Koch has shown, can provide individuals in dire circumstances with resources to manage harsh realities.

Patients are not the only ones who use medicine to manage harsh realities. So, too, do families. In João Biehl's research in Brazil, he has suggested that, in a setting where medications serve as healthcare and infrastructure is defunded and poor, the family serves as the "medical agent of the state, providing and at times triaging care, and medication has become a key instrument for such deliberate action" (2005, 22). Family members make judgments and decisions about sick persons based on a person's adherence to medications, creating and forestalling people's life chances.

I take Biehl's and Koch's observations as a starting point for a further suggestion: the materials and rules of TB treatment (in short, DOTS) offered children a form of agency in their families and a semblance of control within their highly marginalized positions. While researchers of TB, HIV, and other diseases have noted that children can be medicine promoters who encourage adults to take their medicine, my observations propose something much more substantial.[3] Children were taking the rules and materials of treatment and making them their own, using them to shape their relationships to sick adults, their ties to households, and the resources they hoped to receive.

An understanding of children's engagement with global treatment technologies requires some background on the historical changes in TB control measures and how such measures have entered into Zambia and, specifically, George. I start this chapter with a brief history of the increasing pharmaceuticalization of TB.[4] I then describe how DOTS-based practices have shaped TB medication distribution at George Health Centre and are affecting what it means to give good care to TB patients. After providing this necessary background, I will return to the children and show how they were taking the promises of and guidelines on treatment adherence and carrying them out in their homes. I will demonstrate the lengths to which they went and the meanings they associated with adherence. Such an analysis moves us beyond debates about the feasibility of involving children or other family members as observers of TB treatment adherence to an examination of how universal policies and their ideologies transform and become meaningful in local contexts and to particular actors.[5] A focus on children's responses to TB treatment offers unique insight into how global public health technologies can shape and become a resource in children's life projects. In this case, the children followed the rules of treatment to safeguard identities, relationships, livelihoods, and futures that have become increasingly under threat in an era of TB and HIV.

A Brief History of TB Control in Zambia

At Zambian independence in 1964, the new government set out to create a "health service for the people second to none anywhere."[6] This was part of a much larger expectation that Zambia was fast on its way to becoming a modern country with a place in the developed world (Ferguson 1999). TB—a disease that had declined significantly in developed countries by that time—had no place in their vision for their new country. It seemed to officials that, during colonial rule, the Zambian people had not adequately benefited from the pharmaceutical innovations in TB control that had occurred in the first part of the twentieth century.

In the 1920s, the BCG (Bacille del Calmette et Guérin) vaccination was first used in humans to protect against TB and, during the 1940s, effective antimycobacterial chemotherapy was discovered. Both innovations offered a viable means of exporting Western methods of TB control, and officials in Zambia identified these TB technologies alongside improved health services and facilities as the key to eradicating the disease.

To address the TB problem in the new nation, the Ministry of Health and the country's newly created National Tuberculosis and Leprosy Programme (NTLP) launched an ambitious, two-pronged approach: a large-scale vaccination campaign and the isolation and treatment of TB sufferers. The first approach, a BCG vaccination campaign for children, was seen as the route to eradication so that future generations would not develop the disease. The idea was to vaccinate all children in the country through the use of mobile units that could reach even the remotest villages. In 1968, just four years after independence, the Ministry of Health optimistically reported that the country was well on its way to full immunization of children; they had vaccinated one million children around the country.[7] Children were envisioned as the future of a modernizing country, unencumbered by a developing country's disease.

Health officials knew, however, that "[i]t may be some years before the tremendous BCG campaign can be expected to reduce the prevalence of this disease [TB] significantly."[8] They identified their most pressing concern as the numbers of undiagnosed and untreated people with active TB disease. These sufferers were seen as dangerous to the health of the new nation, like "mad men" with shotguns (Richards 1969). Officials viewed this problem as one of access and availability of diagnostic and healthcare services and infrastructure. And, thus, the second approach they initiated to control TB was the active detection and isolation of TB sufferers. They proposed ambitious measures, including mobile TB testing and forced hospitalization:

> We must seek out and find every person in Zambia who is suffering from Pulmonary Tuberculosis. With this aim the Ministry of Health have started a big campaign to X-Ray the chest of every person in Zambia. Mobile X-Ray machines will tour the country, first taking X-Ray pictures of all school children. . . . All persons found to be suffering from Pulmonary Tuberculosis MUST be admitted to Hospital for special treatment. Such people are a danger to the community because they will spread the disease to their relatives and friends. (Richards 1969, 21; capitalization in the original)

Unlike today, TB was not a disease treated on an outpatient basis, but one understood to need isolation. Albert, an elderly man living in rural Southern Province, Zambia, recalled the mobile X-ray units that came to his area and identified him as suffering from pulmonary TB.[9] He was immediately put in isolation in the hospital. Healthcare workers took away Albert's clothes, and would not allow him direct contact with visitors. When family and friends visited, their only way to talk with him was through a grille on the window that separated him from outsiders. Albert and other patients at this time were kept in TB isolation units for three months, and then sent back to their families to continue taking treatment until they completed a twelve- to eighteen-month course.

By 1969, health officials were optimistic about these two TB control measures. Soon after in the 1970s, however, the tenor of the annual Ministry of Health reports had changed as Zambia's economy began deteriorating.[10] Without transportation and other necessary equipment to administer vaccinations, internationally donated vaccine kits remained in storage.[11] Facilities to treat patients were inadequate. Medications were running short.[12] At the end of the 1970s, the Ministry of Health identified that TB was the most pressing cause of death among adults in the country.

Ministry of Health officials could not anticipate what would come in the 1980s and 1990s. To add to the already dire situation that had been mounting with the declining economy in the 1970s, the HIV epidemic took hold in the 1980s, weakening people's immune systems and making them more susceptible to the disease. Structures to manage the emerging crisis were not in place because of the declining economy and neoliberal reforms that were defunding and restructuring the delivery of healthcare. In 1997 Zambia's National TB and Leprosy Programme's external funding agreement with the Netherlands expired and the NTLP nearly collapsed. As a result, the country ran out of TB drugs, and an "unquantified number" of TB sufferers died (Bosman 2000, 606).

The 1990s made an indelible impression on the people who lived through it. Residents of George described this period as a time when, to borrow one woman's words, "you could tell that a person was sick with TB." People's bodies showed visible signs of the disease. They were wasting away, without medical help from the government or external funders, and in a setting where they struggled to keep up with the other aspects of good care for the sick, such as a bed, food, and clean toilet facilities. Residents of George contrast this abandonment—what they called a lack of help—with the government's substantial TB control efforts in the past, after Independence, and also the growing presence of TB medications that have entered the settlement since the turn of the twenty-first century.

A GLOBAL EMERGENCY: THE STANDARDIZATION OF TB PROGRAMMING

The development of a global strategy of TB control solidified biomedicine as the means of TB control in Zambia and elsewhere in the world. By the 1980s and 1990s, Zambia was not the only country facing a mounting TB crisis caused by factors such as HIV, declining economies, and healthcare restructuring.

Recognizing the growing TB burden in many places, the World Health Organization declared TB a global emergency in 1993, a move that drew attention and funding to the disease. One year later, the WHO introduced a global framework for TB management—DOTS—which was based on the research of Karel Styblo, a Czechoslovakian medical doctor and the former director of scientific activities at the International Union Against Tuberculosis and Lung Disease. Styblo dedicated his career to TB control, piloting outpatient treatment efforts using short-course chemotherapy in diverse economic and political locales. The WHO universalized his findings into a five-pronged technological strategy, which has included (1) government commitment to TB control; (2) TB testing through sputum microscopy; (3) standardized and supervised (or observed) medical regimens; (4) an uninterrupted supply of medication; and (5) efficient recording and reporting systems (World Health Organization 1994). Marketed as a universally applicable solution, the introduction of DOTS compelled international interest in TB control, legitimated the intervention of international organizations and funders, and enabled countries to receive financial and technical resources that they could not provide on their own (Koch 2013).

Embedded in the DOTS framework is a fear of "treatment anarchy," the inconsistent access to or usage of TB medications, which can contribute to multi- and extremely drug-resistant TB (World Health Organization 1997). A main tenet of DOTS has addressed patient behavior through a mechanism known as DOT, directly observed therapy. The assumption that underpinned DOT was that direct observation of patients' medication ingestion was a cost-effective and efficient way to replace hospitalization, while still ensuring patient adherence to treatment. In practice, daily contact shifted costs to patients who in some places had to travel for daily or weekly observation while taking their pills, at times causing them to miss work and spend their scarce resources on transportation. Researchers sharply criticized the implementations of DOT for exaggerating patient agency and ignoring the structural conditions that made daily observation difficult or undesirable (Harper 2006; Leinhardt and Ogden 2004).

The mounting critique of DOT prompted a shift in language and practice from punitive to patient centered (Harper 2010). Although initial discussions envisioned the surveillance of daily drug ingestion occurring within health centers, more recent conversations focus on "community contributions to TB care" and "community DOT" (World Health Organization 2003). Public health practitioners increasingly view community health workers as adherence promoters. More patient-centered approaches have included the use of trained community volunteers to visit patients often in their homes (Ayles et al. 2013; Shin et al. 2004).[13] Some researchers have shown that family members might serve as viable treatment supporters (Newell et al. 2006), an idea that has generated some controversy about the role of family in DOT (Freiden and Sbarbaro 2007), even as family members are already playing substantial, informal roles in treatment support.

In George, the mechanisms used to distribute TB medications and monitor adherence represent a bricolage of global, national, and local approaches to managing treatment adherence. Zambia renewed its commitment to DOTS in 2002 after the turbulent period in the 1990s when the NTLP nearly collapsed due to healthcare system restructuring and the withdrawal of external donor funding for specialized TB programming.[14] After the NTLP regained external funding and support, TB focal persons were appointed to government health centers to coordinate TB services according to the DOTS protocol. In George and other clinics serving large populations of TB patients, this restructuring translated into the establishment of TB Corners, physical and temporal locations for distributing TB treatment and monitoring medication adherence.[15] Even though there were a number of private clinics of varying quality in George, the TB Corner at George Health Centre was the only place in George where residents could access free TB treatment in the settlement. Almost every diagnosed TB patient in George ended up in the TB Corner during treatment.

TB TREATMENT ON THE GROUND

The way people move through George Health Centre has everything to do with what ails them. Despite the singularity implied by its name, the clinic comprises eight buildings. Most people find themselves, at least at first, in the oldest and largest building. This building houses examining rooms, a maternity ward, a diagnostic lab, and a pharmacy, among other services. The other seven buildings have been constructed one after another over the past decades with international donor funds and for highly specific purposes: breastfeeding trials, syphilis and gonorrhea research, HIV and AIDS treatment, physical therapy, and, in 2008, TB treatment. In a nod to the verticality of public health programs and the popularity of disease-specific research in urban Zambia (and around the globe), many buildings retain the names of the former projects that funded their construction. Staff working on the Zambia and South Africa TB and AIDS Reduction study, with which I affiliated my research, enjoyed telling people that we could be found in "Breastfeeding," a building constructed for a long-running and completed breastfeeding project carried out by a prominent research university in the United States.

When entering the clinic gate, Breastfeeding is the first building you see. It is located just in front of an older building that contains some offices, a staff cafeteria, and bigger rooms used for different reasons throughout the year. In the rainy season, its biggest room has served as a cholera ward. The driveway branches off between this old, multipurpose building and the main clinic building. At this junction, and during the time of my study, a large sign announced: "Get your *vikolala* [sputum] tested here." A ZAMSTAR worker sat beneath the sign, talking to people about TB testing. Moving straight past the sign, the ARV (antiretroviral) clinic is tucked at the back of the clinic grounds. A left turn at the sign leads to a covered ambulance carport that served as the TB Corner at George Health Centre from 2002 until 2008.[16] The ambulance that once sat in the carport is long gone.

The TB Corner was not simply a space for treatment, but also a practice of treatment. TB drug distribution followed a similar pattern every day. As TB patients and their families filtered into the driveway and carport, the TB Corner nurse and TB treatment supporters, local volunteers trained by NGOs and the District Health Management Team, set up benches and tables. They brought out large containers of TB pills, a hardcover TB Patient Log that listed individual names, addresses, and HIV test results, and a number of paper charts. TB treatment supporters and nurses hurriedly divided pills from large bottles into bags of seven and twenty-eight pills.[17] The patients who came daily for their pills were given a single dose to take at a water station.

Because patients were required to collect their medicine regularly, the TB Corner was packed on every morning of the week, with patients and their family members crowded into the carport and standing along the driveway and grass adjacent the carport. For the first two months, patients were required to collect drugs either daily or weekly. Sometimes, if a person was too debilitated or otherwise unable to come, other household members, kin, or neighbors came instead (a practice that was tolerated to varying degrees by TB nurses). At the end of two months of "intensive" treatment, the "continuation phase" of treatment began, which allowed individuals to collect their medicine monthly.

No Children in the TB Corner

Children were conspicuously missing from the daily bustle of TB Corner activities and TB treatment protocols during my fieldwork in 2005 through 2008, something that has been changing since the World Health Organization placed a spotlight on childhood TB in 2013. Children have not been diagnosed with TB as frequently as adults, for reasons related to the distribution of the disease and the difficulties of diagnosing TB in children, making most patients in the TB Corner older than fifteen. Their accompanying family members appeared just as old and older. Children's absence from the TB Corner seemed to contradict their important and acknowledged role in running errands and responding to the needs of adults, as I discussed in chapter 2. For example, my survey of children's roles across 200 households in George showed that running to stores and tuck shops for medicine such as Panadol (a pain reliever) was a primary errand that many children carried out during the month prior to my survey. Waiting in the TB Corner, however, was an adult errand.

I asked two TB treatment supporters why children in George were rarely sent to the TB Corner to pick up drugs for parents, grandparents, aunts, uncles, or neighbors. Their responses suggested that local concerns over children's risks might have something to do with this rarity:

MAXWELL: We look at the age. Maybe if they're fourteen or fifteen it's okay. But not ten because we restrict. We don't allow children.

JEAN: So if one comes, what do you do?

MAXWELL: We say, "Go and get someone older than you. Here, there is TB here, it can be contracted from here." That's why we don't want children to collect. When we see them, we return them to go and call the "olders" to collect the medicine.

JEAN: Do they ever come back and say that the olders can't come?

GODFREY: No, if they do [come the first time], we do send them [to call someone older]. They do send someone older.

Given the worry over children, if a child was needed to pick up TB medicine from the TB Corner, she was most likely already exposed to the disease in the home. However, the TB Corner demonstrated publicly the possibility of TB infection for everyone. Family members, TB treatment supporters, and nurses sat in poorly ventilated sections of the clinic for long periods of time. Placing a child in such danger, in public, was viewed as unconscionable. TB was an adult's disease and treatment was carried out for and by adults. A view from the TB Corner may suggest that children were not exposed to global ideologies of TB treatment. A household view provides a very different story of children's participation in one of the largest global health efforts in the world.

MAKING CHILDREN'S ROLES VISIBLE

On a hot October afternoon, twelve-year-old Irene rushed toward me as I approached her house, asking: "Did you see my dad at the clinic?" Her usual excitement over my visits was replaced with a tone that conveyed anxiety and fear. Victor and Margrete, Irene's parents, collected Victor's TB medication at the clinic early every Tuesday morning. I had seen them waiting at the TB Corner that morning. However, it was now late in the afternoon and they should have returned. Irene and I stood outside of their mud-brick house with her nine-year-old brother, Floyd, looking in the direction of the health center, a two-kilometer walk on dusty paths that wended their way through tightly packed housing.

While Irene's parents went to the clinic weekly to stand among the crowds of other adults receiving treatment, Irene and Floyd waited at home. They carried out household chores, watched their younger siblings, and generally worried that the clinic visits might indicate their father's worsening condition. That day, Irene and Floyd were selling bags of crushed stones, which Irene had helped her mother crush from a rock outcropping behind their house. Because crushing stones is such hard labor for its payout, this seemed a particularly desperate attempt to raise money to sustain the family. The family members made other last-resort decisions, such as agreeing for their older daughter to marry a man who had impregnated her, a decision that Victor and Margrete had avoided well after the birth of the baby because they were unsure that the union would be in their daughter's best interest. It turned out that it was not. However, the family's financial situation was dire. Both Victor and Margrete had to stop their work, Victor because he was sick and Margrete because she needed to care for him.

As the sun began to set, Margrete returned alone with Victor's medicine. She was angry. Victor had left the clinic hours before after becoming annoyed with the long wait to get both his TB medications and his ARVs. Margrete remained to pick up his medications, without which he would most certainly become sicker. Margrete's disposition changed from anger to concern when she learned that Victor had not returned home. Irene ran out of the house to look for her father and returned thirty minutes later with Victor limping behind her on a clumsy pair of homemade crutches. It had taken him hours to walk the two kilometers on his own. I left as Floyd helped Victor get into bed and rushed to get him drinking water. Irene went outside to cook dinner, and their mother slumped over in exhaustion.

The absence of children at the TB Corner gives a wrong impression of their involvement in TB management and in what the World Health Organization might consider as directly observed treatment. Irene and Floyd's presence at home during Margrete and Victor's weekly trips to the clinic facilitated Victor's TB and HIV treatment and Margrete's ability to give care, while appearing to be separate from it. A simultaneous view of household and clinic provides a more accurate picture of the real work that goes into collecting medicines on such a frequent basis. And it suggests something further, something that the children made evident in their role plays: the clinic and the household are not separate zones of activity. In the children's role plays on "living in a house with a sick person," they emphasized this connection, despite their restriction from clinical space of treatment. Across the nine role plays performed during three separate workshops with different children, all children acted out protracted episodes of walking to and from the clinic to collect medicine. Children demonstrated how the home, the clinic, and the paths in between were implicated in the care and treatment of the sick.

The children's accounts show that "being a TB patient" is a familial—rather than individual—condition. While treatment can be empowering, it is also disciplining. Family members of the sick, as well as the sick, experienced this discipline in their regular trips to get medication from the TB Corner. Children experienced it in their efforts to make these clinic visits possible, through their work in minding smaller children, carrying out household chores or income-generating activities from home, and attending to the sick person, when he or she was left behind, too debilitated to make the clinic trip. As we will see in the following section, the collection of TB medications was not the only aspect of DOTS with which children became involved.

Encouraging Adherence

Global concerns about treatment "adherence" and "default" guide most aspects of TB treatment in George, as they do around the world. Unlike other countries, MDR-TB in Zambia remains low at less than 2 percent (ZAMBART 2011). For the NTLP, this figure situates drug resistance as both a future problem and a very real fear, given the high levels of drug resistance in close-by countries, such as South Africa. The concern over drug resistance is written into DOTS protocol and has led public health actors to recommend patient adherence to drug susceptible regimens as the most important route to averting resistance (Mulenga et al. 2010). The first part of ensuring adherence has been proving and proclaiming its efficacy. The second part is getting patients to take their medicine daily, even when they feel well. The routines around TB treatment in the TB Corner and the innovations of NGOs have served these purposes, while promoting a particular ideology of TB treatment adherence as a community and family responsibility.

Because of the years without treatment, people in George knew firsthand the efficacy of TB medicine and frequently recounted its efficacy, even when it had not benefited their family. I routinely heard that "medicines from the clinic" were what sustained life. TB sufferers and their family members listed home and over-the-counter remedies they used prior to TB diagnoses, but suggested that they stopped these once diagnosed. Prayer complemented biomedical TB treatment, but was not seen as a replacement for it. Only one person in my study admitted to me that she saw a traditional healer during her treatment. Her healer was treating the underlying reasons for all of the diseases from which she suffered, including but not limited to TB. This same woman attended the TB Corner daily.

Even though residents largely believed in the efficacy of TB medicine, not everyone took their medications according to clinical protocol. Taking TB medication was not always easy or possible. Direct observation of treatment had never really caught on in George because debility, distance, and work made it difficult for most patients to come to the clinic daily. Alternatively, resource shortages and the sheer number of TB patients made it impossible for clinicians to bring medicines to patients' houses daily. Clinicians, NGO workers, and local volunteers relied on a range of other materials and activities to promote adherence to medicines. At TB diagnosis, patients were handed their "green card," a folded piece of thick green paper that classified them as a TB patient. Green cards had tiny numbered boxes that patients were asked to tick each time they took their medication for a total of eight months. The nurse reviewed their cards weekly or monthly to ensure that they had not missed a dose. While the cards were the most blatant attempt at monitoring and encouraging adherence, there were many more efforts. Each morning in the TB Corner, activities commenced with a Christian prayer and an educational session, during which the TB Corner nurse, community volunteers, and NGO workers spoke on issues of TB treatment adherence and how to be a good patient and, for family members, how to take good care of a patient. These sessions included explanations of how TB medications worked, with emphasis on the importance of adherence and advice for living a healthy lifestyle.

NGOs working in George experimented with a range of other strategies to enhance adherence to treatment. Alongside the global emphasis on patient-centered TB treatment, their efforts tended to focus on the care needs of patients, and particularly the role of community and family in promoting care. A Japanese NGO known as AMDA-MINDS, for example, trained a set of local community volunteers in George to serve as TB treatment supporters. They helped in the TB Corner, visited patients in their homes, and spread TB treatment messages around the community. The NGO's website explained the TB treatment supporter program in a brief entitled "Zambia: Anti-Tuberculosis Program through Community DOTS in Lusaka Compounds":

> Since TB treatment requires rigid drug adherence and failing to do so leads to a huge risk of producing multidrug-resistant TB, the patients need support from family members and neighbors while coping with social discrimination and stigma. This program is establishing a model to protect communities by the communities. . . . As awareness and understanding on TB among [George] compound residents have been enhanced, and drug adherence has improved, the TB mortality rate has reduced.

In such a perspective, awareness, education, and an encouraging family and community environment, rather than direct observation, were the tools for cultivating adherence.

The twin ideas that TB medications were efficacious and patients needed support and encouragement were encapsulated in graduation ceremonies conducted for people who completed their treatment. AMDA-MINDS supported the graduations as a way to celebrate patients' recoveries from TB, viewing recovery as an achievement facilitated by the clinic, TB drugs, the assistance of TB treatment supporters and family, and an individual's hard work. The graduations were joyous events for the people who attended. However, not one of the eighteen TB sufferers in my study participated in a graduation ceremony. Perhaps the significance of the graduation ceremonies was lost on them because most did not have a TB treatment supporter who regularly visited them. The numbers of TB patients that TB treatment supporters were supposed to follow was large and their efforts voluntary. As a result, TB treatment supporters rarely saw all of the patients they were assigned, and the largest sources of support continued to be family.

While attempts to form a sense of community and accomplishment around TB through graduation ceremonies might have fallen short, the graduations served a less obvious but more significant purpose. Because the building in which they took place was adjacent to the TB Corner, they were conducted in plain view of current TB sufferers receiving their daily, weekly, or monthly allotments of medication. Clinic workers told me that graduation ceremonies provided these people, who were still on treatment at the TB Corner, with the encouragement they needed to keep taking their drugs by acknowledging that others had survived. Encouragement became a strategy used in the TB Corner and beyond to foster both adherence and hope for the future. This focus on encouraging adherence solidified the role of family and community in treatment, whether they were official treatment supporters or not. Children, too, understood and conveyed messages on treatment adherence that came out of the clinic and circulated in their households and community.

"If You Don't Follow the Medicine, You Can Die"

Across my various methods, children emphasized the importance of "following the medication." They used this phrase to refer to taking medicines every morning until treatment completion and also to convey the complex of activities required of patients when on medication. These included attending the clinic, eating a nutritious diet, resting, avoiding strenuous chores or work obligations, and eschewing alcohol and cigarettes. When I asked them about TB in my children's workshops,[18] the children invoked these rules:

> MUSA: If you finish your medication and you start drinking beer you can suffer from TB again.
>
> RHODA: If you are taking TB medication and start feeling better, then if you stop, you won't get better or cured.

Going to a spiritual healer or *nganga* (translated as traditional healer) for TB was not part of the children's understandings of the rules of treatment. When I asked the children if people at times sought care from these other providers, they answered with a resounding "*awe* [no]." In one group, twelve-year-old Irene shifted in her seat after her loud "awe," admitting quietly: "Some people when they have TB they don't come to the clinic, they prefer going to the nganga and [they also prefer] saying that they've been witched. But it's really TB." Repeating widespread public health messages, children suggested that traditional healers who made promises to cure TB or HIV "just want money," "they don't tell the truth," and "they can't heal you." "When you go to a traditional healer," Musa said, "he'll ask for one million *kwacha* and tell you lies." Traditional healers in George acknowledged that biomedicine was the preferred TB treatment option, even for many of them. As one traditional healer phrased it: "When they know that these are TB symptoms, people usually run to the clinic. Unless in those areas where the clinic is far or there is no clinic, then the person will go to the traditional healer first."[19]

In a different conversation, Musa extended this view to the multitude of private clinics that have cropped up in George, and which took his own brother's money while he continued to get sicker. There were extreme consequences for not following the precise rules of treatment or for seeking care outside of the DOTS-organized clinical settings. The children broached these consequences directly in general statements such as: "Not following TB medication, you can die" (Sarafina); "If you don't take the medicine given to you from the clinic, you can die" (Irene).

Chiko took adherence to the rules of TB treatment one step further than other children in my study and, in doing so, showed how family members are also subject to the rules of TB treatment and can be considered adherent or not. One standardized rule of TB treatment is that all pulmonary TB patients in Zambia and elsewhere are required to submit follow-up sputum samples two months into their treatment. This follow-up test, in which patients give sputum three mornings in a row, alerts health practitioners about the efficacy of the medication. If bacilli are not found, it marks a transition from intensive to continuation phase medications and enables a person to collect their medications monthly, rather than weekly. Instead of submitting sputum for her follow-up test, Chiko's mother, Elesia, continued to collect intensive phase medication weekly from the clinic. Elesia told me that it was just too painful to walk so early to the clinic and produce the sputum needed for the test. As Elesia spoke to me about her struggles to produce sputum, Chiko interrupted, telling Elesia that she would give the doctors her own sputum for the test. Elesia's lack of adherence to the diagnostic rules of TB and her continued use of intensive phase medications distressed Chiko as well as her sister, Abby, who wished to usher their mother through treatment to recovery. The delay symbolized a prolonged illness and a looming threat of further separation or their mother's death.

The children's notion of following the medicine offers insight into the powerful juxtaposition of biomedicine, personal and familial responsibility, and recovery. The emphasis that children placed on treatment adherence speaks to the tremendous success of public health campaigns in advancing messages about TB treatment and making medications available. TB treatment held power in children's imaginations because policies that promoted biomedical TB treatment have changed the prognosis of TB for many sufferers. Before viewing children's emphasis on following the rules of treatment simply as repetition of public health messages, we must consider the moral and social assessments and distress in their statements.

Medicine Is Care

Because medicine is equated with cure and there are specific rules to follow to ensure this cure, the practice of following the medicine has become entangled with notions of good family care for TB patients. Recall eleven-year-old Rose's tape-recorded story from the previous chapter, in which she referred to a picture of a person in a hospital bed, surrounded by family members. In her story, she described a father who was sick with TB. Speaking in the voice of the father, Rose said: "I am sick my children. But my children, I am taking my medicine, I went to the hospital and I was given this medicine. In case I might forget my dosage, you should remind me. And they have also given the vitamins. These are the TB tablets. I was also told to eat a lot of food and fruits." In this passage, Rose's father showed himself to be an adherent patient, willing to take his medication and make other adjustments to get well. However, he also suggested that his children had a role to play in supporting his adherence.

Rose's story demonstrates, vividly, how people domesticated the rules of TB treatment in their efforts to show care to loved ones. The process she described was twofold. First, family members showed their care for a patient through helping and encouraging them to adhere to their medicine. And, second, patients reciprocated this care—and showed care themselves—when they made efforts to follow the medicine. At the end of Rose's story, Rose says in her own voice: "He later got better because he followed his medication very well. My father didn't die." This last statement is important because it shows that his death would be indicative of a lapse in care for and by her father, and not a failure of the medication.

Patients invoked the support they received in taking their medication to both express and assess the quality of care they received from family and community members. This became evident in a survey I conducted with TB sufferers during the initial months of their treatment. I was interested in understanding how TB sufferers experienced social support or abandonment, so I asked them to list people who knew about their TB diagnoses and how each person responded to the news of their diagnosis. Munyongo's response to my survey was representative of the majority of responses I received. Munyongo lived alone with her only child, Sarafina. Her husband had died of TB years prior to Munyongo falling ill. While the pair lived alone, they had family nearby in George and also farther away in other residential areas in Lusaka and the rural areas outside of the city. Because she believed that Sarafina was unaware of her TB diagnosis, she did not list Sarafina in her survey response. Here is her list of people who she said knew about her TB and her interpretation of their responses to her diagnosis:[20]

1. [Maternal] uncle: He encouraged me to take the medication and not to miss one dosage of the drug.
2. Elder brother: He also encouraged me to take the medication.
3. Young brother: He also encouraged me to take the medication.
4. Elder sister: She did not want to see me. Even now she does not come to see me.
5. Church members: They encourage me to take the TB drug and they were always visiting me.
6. Cousins: They encouraged me to take the medication and told me that I will be okay.

Munyongo identified encouragement as an act of acceptance. Her elder sister's refusal to come see her was emblematic of a breakdown in the relationship and a lapse in care.

In a similar account, another woman in my study who had TB, Sarah, emphasized her social abandonment in her list. She said that most of her family members "didn't say anything" about her TB when they found out. Only her twelve-year-old niece, Tracy, who moved in to Sarah's house to care for Sarah during her illness said something when she found out about her TB.[21] In Sarah's words: "She encouraged me to take the medicine."

Only people who cared enough encouraged a person to take their medication. In the previous chapter, I suggested that the children's role plays on "living with a sick person" demonstrated children's knowledge of when and where TB was named. I described the role play enacted by Musa (doctor), Rhoda (aunt), Sarafina (mother), and Gift (sick man) as an example. I did not describe how that role play ended. At the eleventh minute, Musa, still playing the doctor, drove his car across the Demonstration Room to where the sick man was living in order to find out why the man was not recovering. The implicit message was that something must be wrong in the family that was preventing the man from recovery. Upon arriving at the house, the doctor learned that the man was living with his maternal aunt and not his mother. The doctor made the following assessment:

> So you, the mother, you want your son to be drinking his medicine from his auntie's place. His aunt won't be reminding him on which time to take the medicine. The aunt won't even care. She'll just be saying, "After all, he's not my

son. That's the reason why his mother chased him [away]. So me I don't care whether he takes his medicine or he doesn't." So just let him take his medicine from here. When he finishes, we'll see how he's going to be.

The tone of the doctor's last sentence was particularly ominous, implying that, even after the man finished taking his medication, he would remain sick because his aunt did not care enough to monitor his medication.

Debates about the proper nurture of the sick often revolved around both the positive and negative sentiments of caregivers, namely mothers, and also the children themselves as caregivers. The children witnessed gendered conflicts in their households and families when sick family members' did not recover quickly enough. These debates occurred during illness and after death. In the role play, Musa, who played the doctor, enacted the debates he witnessed in his own family when his brother moved from his aunt's house to his mother's house. Such debates did not end at death. Particular women, including Musa's mother, received the blame for not monitoring treatment carefully enough. Musa's words offer insight into more than the gender inequalities in care, which I will discuss in more depth in chapter 5. They represented the children's views of their own roles in the care of sick persons and what they perceived as important to ensuring their ill family members' recovery. The children cared enough to make sure that the sick person took their medicine. They accomplished this by remaining close to home.

Adults praised and encouraged children's home-based involvement with medication. When I first met Moffat, a man who suffered from TB and was also on ARVs, he sent his eleven-year-old son, Stephen, to the bedroom to show me his medications. Moffat smiled with pride as Stephen explained when Moffat was supposed to take each pill, showing that Stephen's attentiveness was also meaningful to him. Even if TB did not fit neatly into ideas about childhood, the medicines and rules were available to children. Getting medicine and drinking water not only aligned with DOT, but also fit well with children's socially ascribed roles in households, in which a good child is considered to be one who is responsive to adults. Conversely, a child who does not listen to adults' commands or who stays away too long is considered naughty. It was no surprise, then, that when I asked adults with TB about the changes in their children their most common response was that the children wanted to stay closer to them than before their illness. Staying close was an emotion and practice of care that the children demonstrated through their attentiveness to the sick person's needs. Both children and adults identified the quality of a child's care by invoking the child's proximity and attentiveness, and their willingness to bring TB pills and drinking water for taking the pills.

When the children's parents and guardians became sick, the children positioned themselves to be the family members who reminded them to take their medication. The children showed themselves as particularly knowledgeable about TB treatment adherence and the best ways to encourage and convince someone to take their treatment. Their views are, perhaps, best explained by Abby, Alick, Mulenga, and Agnes in the role play they created on "living with a sick person." All four children were living with an adult who was currently taking TB treatment, two mothers, a father, and a "sister" (maternal relative). In their skit, a young girl's mother, played by Abby, started coughing violently. Agnes, who played the daughter, took a break from washing the dishes to ask Abby: "Mommy, what is the problem? Why are you coughing, coughing? Your cough isn't finishing [getting better]. Do you have a 500 [US$ 0.10] so we can go to the clinic?" Abby handed her daughter the money as Alick, Abby's husband and Agnes's father, returned from work. At the clinic, Abby received a diagnosis of TB and her daughter and husband were given pills. The clinician gave them instructions on how Abby should take them, and he alerted them to watch Abby take them. They returned home, with Agnes keeping careful watch over her mother's medicine. Her concern over her mother's proper use of the medicine culminated in her father attempting to take over her duty of providing the medicine. When Alick motioned as if he were giving medicine to Abby, Agnes yelled: "No, Daddy! It's only one [tablet]!" She grabbed the medication from her father and reinstated her role as the primary treatment observer. The role play continued with Alick playing the clumsy husband and Agnes the knowledgeable young girl in charge of treatment. As opposed to the role play I described earlier, this role play centered on a sick mother. Because of this, the young girl played an especially significant role in caregiving, which included monitoring medicine, a topic I explore in depth in chapter 5.

Children's self-ascribed roles as treatment supporters became most evident during the times when their efforts were constrained. Consider nine-year-old Luka and eleven-year-old Paul's situation. In 2007, Luka and Paul's father, Musonda, started to cough, lose weight, and suffer severe body pains. His legs swelled to twice their usual size, and he could no longer breathe easily. Accompanied by his wife, he made several extended visits to George Health Centre, where he was referred to another health center, farther away from his home, to have an X-ray of his lungs.[22] The X-ray confirmed the suspicions held by Musonda and his family that he had pulmonary tuberculosis.

After Musonda's diagnosis, he and his wife began collecting his TB treatment at the TB Corner. Luka and Paul stayed at home during these clinic visits, but they were in charge of bringing Musonda his medication with a glass of water each morning. It is not easy to take TB drugs when you are sick, and the TB pills are particularly large and difficult to swallow. As Paul once told me, it took particular persistence to get his father to take the medicine each morning when his suffering became too severe, and his father expressed that dying was a desirable alternative.

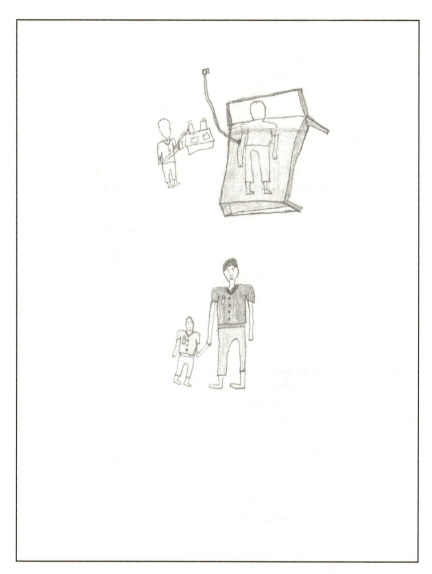

Fig. 4.1 Stephen taking care of his father in the hospital. Stephen accompanies his father on the journey back to George after he is discharged from the hospital. Drawing by Stephen, age eleven.

Six months after Musonda was diagnosed with TB, his condition became so dire that his wife (the boys' mother) took Musonda to the University Teaching Hospital (UTH), the main hospital in Lusaka. From George, UTH is about a one-hour bus trip with a transfer between buses in the city's center. When I heard that Musonda was in UTH, I went there to check on his condition, bring him some food, and see if his wife needed any help. Musonda and his wife were in the male TB ward, a large room with rows of beds. He had been diagnosed with a severe case of pneumonia, but he was given a bed in the ward because he was still on TB treatment. When I left the hospital, I drove to his home in George where I delivered news of his much-improved condition to the children who were waiting at home with relatives who lived nearby. Luka and his brother took my recorder outside and directed messages quietly into the machine. Luka said:

> My dad is in hospital and I feel tired. And since the time he went to hospital, he has not come out. . . . So I asked the doctor if we [Luka and Paul] are allowed to go to [ward number] E21. He said "no." I don't know what to do. Maybe to go through the window? Children are not allowed and the building is tall. So doctor, take care of my father because we won't be coming to see him with medicine every day in the morning before he eats anything.

When I listened to Luka's recording that night, I was struck by his version of adherence, which suggests that children, rather than medical professionals, were responsible for ensuring adherence. In a reversal of clinical roles, Luka told the doctor to attend to his father's medication because "we won't be coming to see him with medicine every day in the morning before he eats anything." Just as the children's role plays showed, caregivers must care enough about the patient to remind them to take their medicine, and the relationship between treatment supporter and patient matters.

Luka's concerns related to his inability to enact care and ensure adherence. Stephen, Moffat's son, expressed similar concerns when Moffat was in the hospital and Stephen was also not allowed to visit. Instead of recording a message, Stephen gave me two drawings made on a single sheet of paper (see fig. 4.1). He described his first drawing: "Daddy is in hospital. He had a problem with the legs and he had a drip of water. I am giving Daddy medicine." In the next drawing, Stephen was holding his father's hand and, in Stephen's words, "Daddy is leaving hospital and he is going home with me holding his hand." I had visited Moffat in the hospital and the scene of the drip and medicine looked strikingly similar to Stephen's drawing. When I asked Stephen how he knew what to draw, he told me that he asked his mother to describe what the hospital looked like. It seems to me that Stephen continued his care for his father, only this time through his drawings. The drawings are a powerful reminder of Stephen's effort to remain present in his father's care when his ability to give care was foreclosed.

TB Treatment and the Category of Child

I have shown in the preceding sections that, in George, DOTS-based programs and the insecurities faced during illness were converging to make observation of treatment (or DOT) a part of what it meant to be a good family member, neighbor, or community member. Children demonstrate that kin and age categories are reinforced, performed, and contested through daily TB treatment. By expressing concerns that relatives, doctors, and other family members might not care enough to encourage or remind their sick parents or guardians, the children were showing that they themselves cared enough. The result was not only hope that a sick person would recover, but also the reinforcement of their belonging in particular households and to particular people.

In chapter 2, I described Musa's experience of being sent to live with a relative on the Copperbelt and how Musa ran back to his mother's care. This was not the first time that Musa took such an approach to his living situation. As a reminder, I first met Musa just after his twenty-five-year-old brother Patrick had been diagnosed with TB and HIV. Following the diagnosis, Musa was sent to live with a relative, whom he called "uncle," a kilometer away. Musa's mother, Judy, reasoned that this move would relieve strain on household resources and protect Musa from TB infection and the burden involved in caring for the extremely ill. Patrick had been the breadwinner for the household, which included six people. Judy was able to make some money by selling hand-knit decorations around George, but she relied on Patrick's substantial inputs. Judy explained to me that they had used all of Patrick's money to seek treatment at private clinics in and around George before he was finally diagnosed with TB at George Health Centre. Plus their rental unit was small, with two rooms, a sitting room and a bedroom just big enough to hold a bed and some shelving. They reorganized their house and daily routines to accommodate Patrick's additional needs. Nights, Judy explained, were the hardest on the household because Patrick had frequent nightmares. When he had to use the outdoor toilet, the entire household woke to clear him a path through their makeshift sleeping areas on the floor and couches and to carry him outside.

To an outsider, Musa's daily life in his uncle's house might have seemed more desirable than remaining in his mother's household during Patrick's care. His uncle was better off than Judy, and he lived in a larger house with leisure items such as a television, radio, and video games. When I asked Musa to draw a day at his uncle's house, he gave me three pages of drawings, in which he presented a detailed account of a day consisting of riding a bike, playing video games, watching a baby, watering the garden, and sitting alone, "just thinking." He was alone most of his days there and had developed a close bond only with one young boy who lived in and carried out work for the household.

After a week in his uncle's household, Musa moved back to his mother's household. According to Judy, he simply showed up and started helping with house chores. I asked Musa why he had returned and if something had happened at his uncle's house to prompt the move. He replied that he needed to help Patrick take his medication.

Patrick did need people to help him take his medicine. He could no longer walk or even sit up on his own. During the last month of Patrick's life, my visits to the household revolved around Patrick's medical regimen. Musa discussed with me the times when they could or could not get Patrick to follow the medication. Patrick was no longer eating, something he needed to do to gain strength and because the clinic rules of treatment emphasized proper nutrition. Patrick's nightmares were worse, which Musa attributed to his medication and actively worked to interrupt by comforting Patrick. Musa slept in the household's only bed with Patrick, stayed near the room during the day, and noticed the smallest changes in Patrick's breathing and movement. Musa's persistence in caring for Patrick legitimated the time he spent with his brother and enabled him to remain in his mother's household, even though he had initially been pushed away.

Musa and other children helped with the medicine because they loved their family members, but their work as medicine supporters should not be considered selfless devotion to family. Instead, I argue that it served as one way in which children attempted to ensure the reciprocal provision of resources and love and preserve their identity as a loved child. Recall in chapter 2 Musa's reasoning for running away from his relatives' house on the Copperbelt. He viewed his mother as an important person who would advocate for his well-being when other relatives might not. His reasoning in that instance is informative for understanding how he interpreted being sent to his uncle's house. In his uncle's house, he risked becoming a child who was in the house but not of the household.[23] This, he noticed, had already happened to the young boy he befriended there, who carried out household chores, but without the reciprocal love and assistance that children typically expect of a good caregiver.

Musa worried that losing proximity to his mother and Patrick would make him an orphan and thereby alter his identity in damaging ways. This loss was more damaging than his potential loss of health. In a different household, as I showed in chapter 3, Chiko became so frustrated when relatives separated her and her older sister Abby from their mother after their mother's diagnosis that she suggested that she and Abby should also get sick with TB so they might be reunited. In this case, the loss of a beloved advocate was viewed as more deadly than the loss of health. The shadow side of the illness of an advocate was the potential social death of the child.

Conclusion

The introduction of universal TB treatment in Zambia has saved lives and demonstrated the efficacy of biomedicine. In its implementation in George, DOTS programming has combined the dual notion that TB treatment must be adhered to and that community and family bear responsibility for adherence. This social side of "following the medication" that has arisen under DOTS and within an overburdened health system is part of a larger pharmaceuticalization of public health (Biehl 2005; Biehl and Petryna 2011) occurring in Zambia where the state's TB management programs now hinge on providing treatment and outsourcing care to families and communities. We need a richer understanding of how such a shift reconfigures social relations, reinforcing inequalities or becoming a tool to redress the harsh conditions produced when poverty and illness combine.

Several aspects converged to shape the ways in which children became involved in TB care: current modes of TB treatment delivery, the needs experienced by households when someone had TB, understandings of what it means to be a responsive child, and children's efforts to create for themselves a good childhood. While TB treatment could be the fault line on which relationships were broken and family members cast out (Biehl 2005), it also represented a resource to negotiate belonging at a time when relationships and futures seemed most fragile. The ways in which the children utilized adherence models suggests that pharmaceutical resources had become indispensable to their efforts to make claims to households, people, identities, and belonging. The children's actions were part of a broader landscape in which community is increasingly experienced and citizenship claims are made on the basis of biology and therapy (Nguyen 2005; Petryna 2002; Rose and Novas 2005). However, the children were experiencing belonging and enacting claims not on the basis of their own biology or therapeutic need, but through attending to the therapeutic needs of loved ones.

Biomedicine is localized in everyday life, its technologies and categories invoked and contested to make sense of experiences of extreme suffering (Ross 2010) and to recast relationships and responsibilities. As João Biehl and Adriana Petryna have observed, "It is at the intersection of the therapeutic imperative, the biotechnical embrace, and the reason of the market that the intensity of survival becomes visible" (2011, 381). The concept of biotechnical embrace, Mary Jo Del-Vecchio Good suggested, implies the affective response associated with biotechnologies. In her words, "'embracing and being embraced' fundamentally links contemporary high-technology medicine and bioscience to the wider society" (2001, 399). The children's embrace of TB technologies became evident in their adherence to rules of treatment, their belief in its efficacy, and the hope it afforded for their futures. TB treatment, because it is so highly effective and requires stringent adherence, shaped their actions and imaginations. And yet, the verb "embrace" is not strong enough. It does not capture the urgency and desperation in their attempts to sustain life, both social and biological.

Over the course of my research, it became clear that the children were neither marginal actors within the national and global programming based on DOTS, nor were they passive victims of the TB epidemic. As TB treatment has become a domestic project within the context of the state's implementation of DOTS, children have also worked to domesticate TB treatment to gain control over, make sense of, and remedy adverse circumstances. Children strategically repurposed TB treatment regimens to reinforce kin relationships and social positions in households. They did this through actions such as reminding loved ones to take medications, showing themselves as knowledgeable about the rules of the medication, and situating themselves close enough to TB patients to administer medication. Carving out their own roles in TB care was an attempt to shape the care, love, and help available to them. This was not an easy task given the transmissibility of TB and the heightened concerns over and reality of children's risks of infection.

Attention to children's roles in TB treatment regimens exposes the forms of life that are forged at the intersection of public health, DOTS, illness, and childhood. As Ross has argued of belonging in a poor settlement in Cape Town: "a life worthy of the name is created by being dependent on others, and that dependence is precarious" (2010, 205). By considering children's roles in TB treatment, we see not just children's dependence, but how some children nurtured dependence through their attempts to create interdependence. The interdependence cultivated by children through TB treatment demonstrates one way in which children engage dominant discourses of global programming, such as DOTS, in resourceful ways that contribute to their sense of belonging to households and kin groups. Such an analysis suggests that the rubric of "treatment support" inadequately captures the meanings of adherence rules for children. Instead, making adherence possible became imperative to cultivating family, community, and childhood under conditions where security in relationships and resources were neither assured nor expected.

CHAPTER 5

Care by Women and Children

Just as my fieldwork in 2008 was ending, I saw Musa's aunt at George Health Centre. We had not seen each other since Patrick's (Musa's brother's) funeral, nearly a year before. At that time, Musa and Patrick's aunt had hosted the days-long mourning service for Patrick at her house on the outskirts of George, where she lived with her husband and four children. I did not immediately recognize her when she shouted my name from across the Health Centre's driveway. She was pregnant and, from her appearance, almost due to deliver. Seeing my confusion, she said: "Jeanie, it's Nomsa, the sister to Amake Musa [Musa's mother]."

Nomsa and I talked about Patrick. She had cared for Patrick in her home during the first months of his illness, when he and the family were still seeking a diagnosis for his worsening health problems.[1] We caught up on other members of Nomsa's family. She asked if I remembered meeting her brother, Alfred, at Patrick's funeral. Alfred's TB, she said, had returned, and he had moved back into her house and into her care, for a second time. Patrick and Alfred were not the only relatives she had nursed during their TB illnesses. As she and her sister repeated often, the disease ran through their family; one of their relatives died from TB every year.

Nomsa was not at the clinic that day to collect her brother's TB medication. And she was not there for a prenatal visit. Instead, she was there to get ARVs for a little girl whose parents—also Nomsa's relatives—had died shortly after Patrick. This little girl, like many family members before her, now lived with Nomsa and depended on Nomsa's care. As part of that care, Nomsa regularly carried the child several kilometers to the clinic to receive treatment for HIV from George's ARV Clinic at the Health Centre. Because of the advanced stage of her pregnancy, however, Nomsa could no longer carry the girl. Nor could she afford the cost of the taxi fare to get the child to and from the clinic. As a result, the little girl stayed home and Nomsa's young children kept watch over her. Nomsa walked alone to the clinic to meet with the little girl's nurse and collect her ARVs.

The struggles Nomsa faced in keeping up with her family's care needs, alongside of her own need for care, may seem extraordinary. Recall, however, that Nomsa's sister, Judy (Musa's mother), faced similar caring responsibilities as she cared for her sick husband, her brother, her grown son and daughter, and her young children. Since the 1980s, this burden of care has become the norm for women, rather than the extreme, as a result of the HIV epidemic. HIV has severely stretched economies of care, and it overshadows all aspects of women's caregiving and care seeking. As I spoke with Nomsa at the clinic entrance that day, I wondered: If Nomsa became sick, who would care for her? My observations of Nomsa's family and of many families throughout my years of living in Zambia have affirmed that children assume much household and nurturing work. A primary goal of this book has been to make children's care as visible in the literature on illness and caregiving as it is on the ground.

In this chapter, I offer detailed ethnographic accounts of children's care for and by sick women. I situate these ethnographic accounts in a long tradition of medical anthropology research in Africa that has attended to the social and familial basis of illness management.[2] This rich body of scholarship has made evident that social hierarchies and vulnerabilities affect the types of treatment people receive during illness, and can lead to unequal treatment and even social abandonment. Scholarly examples of abandonment of the sick have highlighted gender inequalities in care, in particular.[3] Such work, together with my own observations that children take up much care work for women, raises questions about how children, in particular, figure into processes of illness management, including social abandonment. I focus on two separate cases. I first discuss Sarah, a mother of three, who relied on her own children and her niece for care during her illness. Second, I turn to another mother, Munyongo, who lived alone with her young daughter. Without an intimate understanding of the relationships between women and children, both cases I describe seem to convey breakdowns in kinship care—the kinds of breakdowns that are invoked often in research and policy documents to describe the strains on family resources caused by poverty, HIV, and current treatment contexts. The cases do, in fact, make evident institutional and social failures. They lay bare gendered inequalities and violence that have rendered TB deadly for women.[4] Yet, as I will demonstrate, the women in these two cases were working hard to retain kinship ties—and a sense of normality and social value—during their illnesses. Their children proved key to their efforts. The contributions of this chapter are, in part, in the detailed examination of how and to what ends some women and children were creating relationships and solidarities within nearly impossible situations. My contributions are also methodological, reinforcing my argument throughout this book that we cannot understand how social forms and relations change within epidemics without considering children.

GENDER AND CARE

To twenty-nine-year-old Sarah's neighbors in George and outside observers such as myself, Sarah's household appeared relatively well-off for the area. Sarah lived in a new three-room house with her husband and children. The house was tucked behind older, rundown houses along a narrow dirt road, where Sarah and her husband, Friday, built it in 2005. The house was fashioned from cement bricks and had fresh coats of white and blue paint, a metal roof, and glass windows with burglar bars—luxuries by most accounts in George. Sarah believed, correctly, that her neighbors envied her good fortune. Neighbors spoke with suspicion about the quick construction of the house, gossiping that Sarah and Friday must have used illicit strategies to get the money to build it. To add to neighbors' gossip, Friday fell ill with TB shortly after the house's construction. In 2007, when Sarah was diagnosed with TB, she knew that her illness would provide still further commentary on the household, and so she worked hard to hide her illness and to avoid particular neighbors.

Sarah's household offers an example of the gendered struggles over resources and care that occur in households in Zambia.[5] Sarah and her husband, Friday, did not pool their earnings and Sarah did not know how much money Friday earned through his various jobs.[6] By day, Friday was a carpenter. However, he made most of his money from buying and selling televisions and pool tables. All Sarah knew was that this latter work proved lucrative and funded both the construction of the house and the purchase of a taxi, which was to be another source of income, except that Friday wrecked it during a late-night drinking binge soon after he acquired it. Because Friday paid for the construction of the house, he claimed sole ownership. His name alone was on the title deed, and Sarah was treated as a visitor in the house, who could only stay as long as she was welcomed.

For the years I have known Sarah, she has had to find ways to sustain herself and her children because Friday rarely contributed to food, clothing, or the children's school fees. Before she became sick with TB, Sarah supported herself and the children with earnings she made from her informal charcoal business. She walked to rural areas to buy large bags of charcoal that she then sold in smaller quantities to neighbors and passersby. She made these walks with decreasing frequency during the months it took for clinicians to diagnose her TB. As her illness progressed, she spent her needed capital on taxis to clinics, X-rays, and medicines for a variety of ailments, and before long, Sarah had to stop her business altogether.

Aware of her struggles, Sarah's father offered to give her the money she needed to start a new, less taxing, business. The money would have changed her situation, Sarah told me. But Friday refused her father's money, saying that her father was not her husband, and that he, instead, should give her the money to start a new business. Distressed when this did not happen, Sarah complained to me that Friday did not buy her "so much as a panty." He instead spent money on his pregnant girlfriend. She continued to say that he did not pay for the children's school fees or food, and he ate luxury foods, such as sausages, in front of their hungry children. Sarah read the lack of money he spent on her and the children—and the amount of money spent on his girlfriend—as a commentary on their marriage. She both dreaded and dreamed that their marriage would end. In her dreams, she would start over with a new, kinder husband, who would share his earnings with her, giving her the means to invite me and other visitors to her home for tea, "as a Mrs. should." Sarah hated that she could not make food for visitors in her current situation and desired the social status and sentiments that serving food to company could cultivate. At the same time that Sarah dreamed of life untethered to Friday, she dreaded leaving him. She doubted that her life could be as she dreamed. Plus her difficulties in leaving Friday were many. Similar to many women in George, Sarah had to pay careful attention to her marital and familial relationships to retain her social standing and identity.

Sarah's worries about a life without Friday, and without her children, were at the forefront of her mind during her illness. At this time, Friday was actively working to get Sarah to move out of his house. He used many means to get her to leave him or her family to take her in because he knew that divorcing Sarah would cost him money in court. He was abusive. He made claims that Sarah did not uphold her marital duties. He met with Sarah's father and other relatives to complain that Sarah did not clean the house like a good wife should. According to Sarah, he wanted her out so that his much younger and healthier girlfriend could move into the home.

Sarah could not bear separating from her children. In Sarah's understanding, leaving her children would affect the children's life chances. Sarah also expressed how much she would miss her children if they were separated from her. Family members and friends advised her to stay with Friday, both for the children and for herself, even when they knew the depths of her troubles. They told her he might change, words that held weight for Sarah because, despite everything, she deeply loved him. Sarah's troubles remind me of a statement made by Ann Schlyter, a longtime researcher in George, who has written about gendered inequalities in the residential area. She has observed, "The body is an important resource around which women strategise their life course. The first challenge is to stay healthy and alive and to do so, they have to negotiate their sexuality, fertility and family relationships" (2009, 32). Sarah shows that these are not concerns that stop when women become ill, though they become even more challenging and also direr for women to manage.

Then just when Sarah started recovering her strength in 2008 and again considered divorcing Friday, this time with the means to support her children, Friday fell ill. He suffered a recurrence of TB and was diagnosed, eventually, as having HIV. Sarah had watched and commented on his coughing and dramatic weight loss for weeks as he ignored her suggestions to go to the clinic. She knew it was TB but she could not compel him to seek a diagnosis. When his condition became so bad that family members made him go to the clinic against his wishes, his diagnostic and treatment experience bore little resemblance to hers. While Sarah endured the long walk to the clinic alone when she was sick and had to use her remaining savings for taxis, Friday went to the clinic with relatives and in a borrowed car. Friday received money and food to help him recover more quickly. Kin on both sides expected Sarah to accompany him and to nurse him back to good health. As a result, Sarah could no longer enact her plan to leave. She did not want to leave, either. Friday's illness made him a kinder, more grateful man, adding to her hopes that he would change into the loving husband of whom she dreamed.

Sarah and other wives in my study placed extraordinary emphasis on care for sick husbands and on providing visible acts of nursing. They nursed men for reasons related to love, obligation, and reciprocity, and also to avoid the judgment of others, particularly kin. As Frederick Klaits has shown in Botswana, the high demand on women to nurse the sick and provide other forms of labor and care within the HIV epidemic has "focused popular attention on the love (or lack thereof) with which women undertake such work for particular persons in particular places" (Klaits 2010, 17). Where caregiving capacities were not just in high demand, but where women were judged for the quality of their care, women must provide care as a means of avoiding the suspicion or blame of onlookers. They provided care, also, to retain desired and normative identities and family relationships as well as access to housing and resources. Even though Friday did not regularly share food or money with Sarah and their children, Sarah had a level of security and social standing as wife and mother in Friday's house that she did not believe existed for her outside of it.

Friday's fragile bodily state provided welcome respite for Sarah from Friday's abuse and absences. Prior to his illness, he spent most days and nights away from home, and with his girlfriend. However, during his illness, he stayed close to home to receive Sarah's care and affections. Friday's actions and presence made her think back to the comments people made about his ability to become a good husband, and she worked to cultivate loving sentiments between them. She was able to show him love and care through her nurturing role that she could not when he was healthy and spending time with his girlfriend. Her efforts validated her position as his wife, and he expressed appreciation and love for Sarah in his weakened state. She hoped her care might transform their relationship and his treatment of her in the future, something that has not ultimately happened, though they were still married when I visited their home in 2014.

Sarah's children were critical actors in her efforts to strategize her life course, especially during her illness. Recall that Sarah could not move out of the house to receive care from relatives because of her fear of losing her children. As a visitor in Friday's house, she was also not able to have relatives visit to give care to her, without causing a rift in her relationship with Friday. This caused a dilemma for Sarah and her extended family as to how to best care for Sarah when she was sick. In the following section, and through Sarah's case, I will show that children were able to enact nurturing tasks for women that other kin could not, either because other kin were unavailable to give care or an adult's caregiving would be disruptive to a woman's status as wife or mother.

"She Is My Mother"

I was first introduced to Sarah in August 2007, when she received her TB diagnosis. We met at George Health Centre. She had come to the clinic alone, wearing a dress made of colorful *chitenge* fabric.[7] She hoped the chitenge dress would disguise some of the more obvious signs of her illness: her too-thin body and pallid skin. Sarah had spent months trying to get a diagnosis for symptoms that progressively worsened and were—on the day we met—finally labeled as TB.

On that same day, Sarah had spoken with staff working on the Zambia and South Africa Tuberculosis and AIDS Reduction study. They had asked her if she was interested in participating in their research. When she adamantly refused their study, a member of the study team called my cellphone and suggested that I come to the clinic to meet with her because she had children living in her home. He doubted that she would be interested in my study, though he thought I might as well ask her. Perhaps Sarah was too tired to set off in the heat for her long walk home but, for whatever reason, she was still at the clinic when I returned and she listened to me explain my study. After I finished, she appeared wary and nodded her head. She had a baby daughter and ten- and six-year-old sons. She said it was good that I was talking to children (as opposed to adults): "My [oldest] son will tell you many things about our life that I will never admit." She told me to come to her house the following day to ask her children if they were interested in participating in my study.

Sarah's decision to take part in my study while refusing to participate in the ZAMSTAR study seemed contradictory, at first, but it became highly logical in retrospect. ZAMSTAR's focus on medical testing might negatively affect her marriage and consequently a range of other relationships, particularly her relationship with and claims to her children. My study was different. I was not

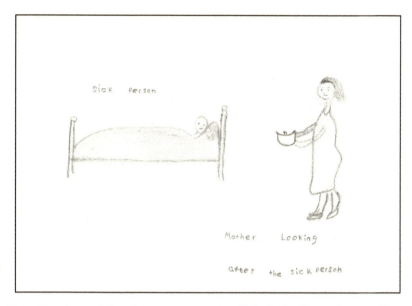

Sick   Person

Mother   Looking

after   the   sick person

Fig. 5.1 Drawing made in reference to my question: "Who looks after a sick person?" Stephen drew a woman bringing food to a sick man. He wrote: "Mother looking after the sick person," identifying the social expectations that mothers care for the sick. Drawing by Stephen, age eleven.

carrying out biomedical tests, in particular an HIV test, which might alter her social status and social relations. Sarah betrayed her suspicions that she and Friday had HIV, making comments about bodily conditions as signs. As the first in a relationship to receive a positive test, she would be the first to receive blame, which could set off a potential chain of other negative events and affect her marriage, kin relationships, and claims to her children. Instead, my research affirmed her status as a mother in contrast to her status as a TB patient and validated her role in her children's lives. My clear focus on children aligned with Sarah's interest in nurturing and remaining close to her children in spite and because of her TB diagnosis.

On my visit to Sarah's house the day after I met her at the clinic, Sarah emphasized again that the children did everything for her. No one else helped her. Her comments indexed two facts about her life: first, the lack of care she received from her husband and, second, the death of her mother years ago. Her mother, she recalled, never wanted Sarah to marry Friday. If her mother had lived, she would have seen that things between Sarah and Friday had turned out the way she had anticipated: very poorly. Sarah's mother would have stood up for Sarah, either taking her in or staying in her home, and she would have cared for her in ways that other kin could not. Sarah rarely cried in front of people, but speaking

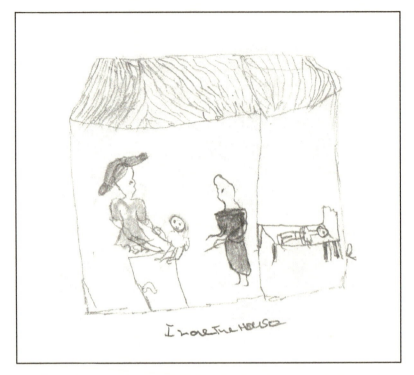

Fig. 5.2 Tracy taking care of Sarah and Sarah's baby when Sarah was sick. Drawing by Tracy, age twelve.

of her mother at that time made tears stream down her face. Her one-year-old daughter reached up and wiped them away.

As Sarah's daughter touched Sarah's face, I considered the severity of the situation. Sarah sat her daughter on her lap and pointed to her twelve-year-old niece Tracy, who sat on the couch with Sarah's sons. Sarah switched from Nyanja to English, and shouted: "Jean, she is my mother!" I had not known that Tracy was living with Sarah at the time, and I was still unsure how Sarah and Tracy were related. I also did not know how to respond to her statement, so I followed with a question about their relatedness. Realizing that I had missed her point, Sarah repeated: "She is my mother." I watched Tracy's amusement and Sarah's stead-fastness. Tracy, she said, did everything that her mother would have done had she been alive. She moved to Sarah's home when she became sick, nurtured and protected Sarah, made sure that she ate and took her medicine, and shared in the household chores. Tracy—Sarah's sister's daughter—even cared for Sarah's baby as if the baby were her grandchild. I read gratitude in Sarah's emphasis on all of the things that Tracy accomplished for Sarah, including giving the impression to Friday and outsiders that Sarah was keeping up her duties as wife and mother.

Sarah's reframing of her relationship to Tracy offered a return to recognizable forms of care between a mother and daughter in Zambia, which were necessary for her return to health (see fig. 5.1). I find Julie Livingston's (2005) historical and ethnographic view into women's caregiving in Botswana helpful for understanding the weight of Sarah's emphasis on her mother's absence and, then, on Tracy as her mother. Women, Livingston writes, were and continue to be "specially positioned within the world of care," and "(m)otherly love, infused with the special qualities of a woman's heart, was a basic and essential attribute seen as necessary for life, health and caregiving" (2005, 99).

Tracy was not just a mother; she was a borrowed child. In chapter 2, I showed some ways in which people in George attempted to solve problems of poverty and related issues through lending and borrowing children. Tracy's move was, in part, an act that demonstrated, and strengthened, the ties between households, as has been shown in a range of Africanist scholarship on the value of children.[8] But it was more than this. Tracy's move was indicative of the lengths Sarah's family, and Sarah's sister in particular, had to go to care for Sarah, including acts of subterfuge. The stated reason why Tracy was there was to visit, not to care for, Sarah. Neither Sarah nor Sarah's sister could move out of their households without damaging their relationships or neglecting their obligations to their husbands and children. In this and other cases, children like Tracy became part of the flexible ways in which women cared for one another, when their caregiving capacities were stretched or denied. Specifically, Tracy was to care for Sarah when no other maternal relatives could do so given the constraints of Sarah's marital relationship. Tracy was sent into a situation where Sarah's husband would not have accepted another woman caregiver and where Sarah's move away from the household could be read as the end of her marriage. The timing of Tracy's move corresponded with Friday's complaints about Sarah's housekeeping as well. It seemed that her move into the house was the family's indirect and discrete response to his complaints and to Sarah's situation and needs.

Tracy's mother coordinated and in certain ways benefited from Tracy's move to Sarah's household, and Tracy was happy to help her aunt. Tracy adored Sarah and Sarah's children, whom she had visited in the past but never for so long. She illustrated her life with Sarah in positive ways, writing "I love this house" and "I love this family" over drawings of Sarah's house, Sarah, and Sarah's children. In one of her drawings (fig. 5.2), Tracy depicted herself helping Sarah with the baby while Sarah was sick. Friday appeared in the drawing only as a figure asleep in the bedroom. In fact, Friday was absent during much of the time Tracy was there. When he was home, in stark contrast to his wife, he viewed Tracy as a burden on the household. He claimed that Tracy was eating their food "as if she does not have a father," an assertion that suggested that Friday was unwilling to stand in as a father to a girl whose parents were still alive. When Sarah told him that Tracy helped out, he said that Samson, their ten-year-old son, was capable of accomplishing Tracy's chores. Sarah did not view Samson's and Tracy's care as interchangeable, and she was not so willing to accept her husband's substitution because of what it might mean for her as a mother.

Managing Motherhood

Though Sarah would never consider Samson "her mother," as she did Tracy, she recognized him as a caregiver. Whenever I visited the house during the first months of her illness, he was carrying out chores or waiting to run errands, or he was sitting next to her on the couch, comforting her and keeping her company. He pleaded with Sarah to attend church gatherings every afternoon and she listened. This was something that Sarah did not do before falling ill, but made herself do in response to Samson's pleas. Months later, after Friday set fire to Sarah's clothing in a fit of rage, Sarah was able to draw on her relationships with women in the church for material support. She credited Samson with cultivating these connections. Ultimately, however, Sarah was clear that her relationship with Samson and her other children centered on a different form of relatedness, one in which she emphasized her motherhood, including her responsibility to protect them. Even as Sarah needed motherly love to return to health, she would be judged against the ideals of motherly love she provided for her own children (Livingston 2005, 99).[9]

The necessity of enacting motherly love became explicit a couple of months into my research with Sarah. I was still uncertain about some details of Sarah's quest for therapy and the family's management of her illness. I thought such issues might be better explored in all of the households through a semi-structured interview with the person who was ill. My aim was to record details that led to TB diagnosis such as treatment seeking and the roles of various kin in offering advice, assistance, and support. I wanted to know about what transpired after diagnosis, and I was particularly interested in learning about stigma, disclosure, and social networks. Sarah and most other women in the study had plenty to say about each of these questions.

When I asked a second set of questions about how the women's illnesses had affected their children, however, most women's demeanors changed. I compiled the latter questions based on recent research, claims in the media, anecdotal accounts I heard from aid workers and community members, and my own observations during the study. I asked about changes in children's behavior, well-being, and roles: Have the children started obeying you more; have they started disobeying you more; are they missing more school than usual; have their grades dropped; have they started doing more piecework or other types of work outside the home; do they carry out more household chores than they used to; have their diets changed (and how); have they stopped playing with their friends; and are they experiencing gossip because of your illness?

By this point in the research Olivious and I had become regular visitors in Sarah's home. We spent dusty, hot season afternoons lounging with her and the children on the couches in their sitting room, watching soap operas and chatting. Sarah had already mentioned the tremendous care she received from the children, and we had witnessed the children's efforts to care for Sarah. Sarah's early guardedness had fallen away to expose a dry- and quick-witted woman with a strong sense of humor. But when I started to ask her questions about her ten- and six-year-old sons, she became defensive, answering with a resounding "no" to each question we asked.[10] Sarah seemed to suggest that there were no changes at all in the children's behavior, activities, and everyday lives since she became ill. This line of questioning embarrassed her. And I felt terrible for creating such palpable discomfort.

In looking back on these questions, I recognize that they revolved around the central themes of children suffering, adults not providing for children, and children not offering enough care or love. I was asking about a breakdown in sociality and social obligations, something that most women and children were struggling against. My questions, which seemed benign before I took Sarah through the questionnaire, were in effect calling into question her ability to mother her children properly. Many other women responded to my set of questions about children living in their households in ways that resembled Sarah's response, often deflecting further inquiry by emphasizing that everything had remained the same.[11]

Had Sarah answered "yes" to the questions, she would have suggested that her poor health affected her ability to properly care for and show love to her children. Recall that Friday was already talking to relatives about the way she kept the house, which had compelled Sarah's sister to send Tracy. He had also criticized Sarah's ability to mother. Sarah was unable to keep her children in their expensive private schools after she stopped selling charcoal. She transferred Samson from private school to the nearby government basic school. Friday was also threatening to entrust one of their sons to relatives who lived outside of Lusaka. Just weeks after I administered the questionnaire and against Sarah's wishes, Friday managed to send their six-year-old son to his relatives' home in Livingstone, a town on the southern border of Zambia.

The women who were ill admitted to children's household work and care for two reasons: to indicate a child's love and attachment to them and as a commentary on the lack of other social systems of care. While references to children's care indicated the direness of their situations, women noted children's efforts with gratitude. For example, Maureen, the mother I mention in the opening pages of this book, told me repeatedly that Loveness and Bwalya were taking good care of her. Women such as Maureen and Sarah often balanced comments about children's caregiving with descriptions of the ways in which they gave reciprocal care to children. Children's caregiving created a moral crisis for women. While the presence and productive labor of children made women's return to everyday life possible (as children kept up with household chores and assisted with nurturing and treatment), children's caregiving also threatened that return to everyday life. When children provided too much, women were seen and also saw themselves as not sufficiently caring for children—as not sufficiently mothering.

Children were aware of this bind for women and themselves. One result was that children made explicit attempts to demonstrate how they received care from women, particularly mothers, during a woman's illness. For example, when I asked Alick to draw a picture of how he gave care to his mother, he drew his mother helping him out of a tree in which he was stuck, an activity that she was not physically capable of doing. Rather than misunderstanding the exercise, Alick wanted to show that his mother helped him when he needed her. The children's positioning of women as their caregivers related to their view that their well-being and futures depended upon women—and not men. Even when children's resources came from men, they were distributed, typically, by women, and children saw women as key to gaining access to men's resources.

Women were advocates and also the gatekeepers to food, shelter, and other resources that children needed. Sarah's case has provided but one example. In the following case, I offer a different view into women's and children's struggles to survive and retain their futures during a woman's illness. While Sarah's case showed the difficulties and tradeoffs involved in drawing on kin during illness, the following case of Munyongo demonstrates how avoidance of kin served as a direct attempt to preserve relationships and manage identities for herself and her daughter, in the present and for their futures.

AVOIDING KINSHIP CARE

On a scorching October day, thirty-three-year-old Munyongo stepped outside of her home, sat down on the stoop, and began washing the laundry her daughter had left in a large plastic basin. It was the first day in months that her neighbors had seen her outside for such an extended period of time. Even though I had known her for two months, it was the first day that I had ever seen her out of her house.

Munyongo and her daughter lived in a one-room unit at the end of a long corridor, and so my first cues that she was feeling better came from other people. I had passed Sarafina, Munyongo's nine-year-old daughter, at a shallow well on my way to their house. She was unusually animated when she called to me from the well. As I approached the housing units where Munyongo and Sarafina lived, several neighbors shared complicit smiles and nodded their heads down the corridor to where Munyongo was sitting, with her back to us. Hearing me greet her neighbors, Munyongo turned her head. I must have had a look of concern on my face, because the first thing she said was: "Sarafina is very much committed with these chores. This is too much for a small child. I need to help her." Though Sarafina took over the washing when she returned from the well, the effort made by Munyongo was significant.

During the weeks prior to this visit, Munyongo had always been in bed when I arrived, with the door to their one-room house slightly ajar and Sarafina inside or nearby. Sarafina would pull out chairs for Emily and me, and then disappear behind the bed sheet that divided their single-room home into two living spaces: a bedroom and sitting room. Each time I visited, Munyongo slowly emerged from the other side of the sheet, walking with agonizing precision and pain. She would then fold her slight body onto the floor. During those visits, Emily and I talked to her about her struggles with treatment and other topics, but mostly we sat quietly with her until she needed to return to bed.

Throughout the initial months I knew Munyongo and Sarafina, I considered the pair to be a most extreme case, exemplifying a collapse in kinship mechanisms of support. I was not alone in my concern over the severity of their situation. A clinic volunteer who knew of Munyongo and Sarafina had set up our first meetings with Munyongo. The two were all alone, he told us. They needed support because Sarafina was doing all of the chores and looking after her mother. Munyongo's husband had died, and there were no family members helping them.

Munyongo spoke with regret about the effects of her illness on Sarafina's workload and schooling. She had transferred Sarafina from an expensive, all-day private school to the nearby government school. The school was not just low cost; it also had much shorter school days, which allowed Sarafina to spend more time at home. And yet at her sickest, Munyongo never wanted Sarafina to miss a day of school, regardless of how greatly she needed her help while she was gone. The dates in Sarafina's school notebook confirmed, too, that she spent much more time at school when her mother was the sickest, and only started missing school when her mother returned to work.[12] Sarafina's thoughts on schooling are informative here. She gave me the following commentary in response to a drawing of a schoolboy that I showed her:

> Children like going to school. When going to school they carry their bags with clean shoes and clean uniform. On their way to school, they stop and start playing with their friends. At 17:00, when some of their friends at school knock off they go home together. When talking to their parents, they lie saying we went to school but if their parents ask for their notebooks, they refuse, saying we didn't write anything today because the teacher didn't come. So parents talk

to teachers for pupils to be knocking off at 17 hours and to take them to school
until they are in class.

In this quote, Sarafina suggested that parents make children go to school. Sarafina
never questioned whether or not she would go to school when her mother was
sick. Going to school during these times was part of her care for her mother and
a way for her to show her love. Sarafina hated her new school, but she shielded
her mother from these feelings while her mother was sick. Going to school not
only pleased her mother; it enabled her mother to mother her, if only through
bedside requests.

When Sarafina was not at school or drawing water from the nearby well, she
remained at home, close to her mother's side. Weeks passed and Munyongo
slowly began walking and assisting Sarafina with the household chores. Sarafina
often took over these activities in ways that did not draw attention to Munyongo's
weak bodily state. Neighbors helped Sarafina draw water or collected medicine
for Munyongo. The absence of Munyongo's kin during her illness increased the
community's imperative to accompany both Munyongo and Sarafina.[13] It induced
comments from neighbors and clinic workers about the pair's dire situation. The
people who made such comments could only do so much to help. They were
dealing with their own crises of care and, more than anyone else, Sarafina provided Munyongo's care needs. Yet even while Munyongo relied on her daughter,
she made attempts to care for her. During the worst of Munyongo's illness, Munyongo's care for her daughter showed through in small ways, and then in bigger
ways as she recovered.

Throughout the early months of her illness, I and the treatment supporters at
the clinic assumed that Munyongo had no family remaining either in or outside
of George. It took me off-guard then when I learned that Sarafina wanted badly
to visit family during the Christmas school holiday. Her desire to leave for holiday surprised me even more given the close proximity she kept to her mother. As
the holiday approached, Sarafina announced to me, with disappointment, that
she would not go on holiday because her mother needed her in the home. Nevertheless, a week later, she was across Lusaka, visiting her mother's brother and his
family. Munyongo framed Sarafina's visit in this way: "I decided that she had to
go because she usually never gets to go on holiday these days." She discussed it as
a break for Sarafina and framed this break in terms of the tremendous care Sarafina provided her and the sacrifices that Sarafina had made. But there was more.

As I described in chapter 2, holidays provided flexible times when children
could get to know relatives, receive and give support, reaffirm normative identities, and much more. Munyongo and Sarafina were both aware of Munyongo's
fragile health and the eventuality of Munyongo's death. Holiday seemed to fit
in with Munyongo's and Sarafina's broader tactics to maintain and cultivate ties
that Sarafina would eventually need to draw on. Notably, Sarafina's holiday visit

was not about Munyongo's illness. It was about Sarafina as a school-going child, spending time getting to know, rather than being supported by, her relatives. As one of the only signs of familial support to the household during Munyongo's illness, this visit was suggestive of how Munyongo and Sarafina strategized care for themselves and each other through deliberate avoidances.

When Munyongo became well enough to return to work, I started meeting a number of family members who came to Munyongo and Sarafina's house. They came from their own houses nearby to watch TV with Sarafina while Munyongo was away at work. Where, I wondered, were they when Munyongo was so sick? Munyongo and Sarafina gave us piecemeal information about their family. Before becoming sick, Munyongo had nursed a sister who had suffered and, later, died from TB. Munyongo associated her TB with the nursing care she gave to her sister, something that she alluded to with resentment in peripheral comments about the transmissibility of TB. Her sister died during the first few months of Munyongo's illness, which may have indicated how much of a crisis her extended family was facing when Munyongo fell ill.

Munyongo was not entirely abandoned by her family, though. I learned that a rural relative had come to George to take care of Munyongo when she heard that she was sick. Munyongo, however, sent the relative away. She gave little information about why she did so. One possible reason could be that receiving assistance from kin typically entails reciprocation, as anthropologist Carol Stack (1974) has suggested in her work on kinship among African American city dwellers in the midwestern United States. Munyongo's steady wage labor allowed her to maintain distance from ties that many women's (and men's) economic activities did not. It also kept her extremely busy. Her initial response, when we met, was to decline my study because of her busy schedule. In her extremely fragile state, she advised me that she was not going to be able to spend any time with me. Given her situation, perhaps it was more desirable to avoid the return claims on her time, caregiving capacity, and money. Her plan to return Sarafina to an all-day private school and provide her with her needs seemed to require the avoidance of such a debt.

Illness and Entrustment

Only in retrospect is it evident how some of the strategies employed by Munyongo and Sarafina actually kept intact additional kinship ties that Sarafina, in particular, might need in the future. The importance of these ties to both Sarafina and Munyongo became apparent upon Munyongo's return to relative health. When Munyongo had recovered from the worst of her illness, she gave Sarafina a princess-themed party for her tenth birthday at her grandparents' home nearby. Sarafina proudly showed me the photographs they took during the party. Her hair was freshly plaited and she wore a frilly pink dress and tiara. There was a cake and dancing. A number of extended family members gathered around for the festivities. In this instance, Sarafina's position was enviable. I knew of no other children who received such a birthday celebration. It was a symbolic gesture that at once demonstrated Munyongo's love for Sarafina, affirmed her abilities to take care of her daughter, enacted a particular idealized version of childhood, and showcased Sarafina as a young girl who was loved, and thus deserving of love and care, even in the event of her mother's death. Munyongo acknowledged the wider family by inviting them to participate in the celebration and the food and drinks that she provided. To be sure, these were luxuries in George. Through Sarafina's party, Munyongo demonstrated an investment in her daughter and, equally important, her relationship with the family members who might someday care for Sarafina.

In certain ways, Munyongo acted to preserve kin ties during her illness by not drawing on them, forestalling feelings of resentment that might have arisen during her prolonged care, such as the ones that Munyongo and her family felt toward her deceased sister. I have heard people in George refer to the negative effects of resentment, jealousy, and HIV stigma, related to parental illness, on children's well-being after parents die. Feelings of resentment and the knowledge that a parent died from AIDS-related causes, people said, affected the care that children receive from exhausted and already overburdened relatives. Munyongo hinted at this when she described her sister's death and the children that her sister had left behind.

In research on women's residential decisions in South Africa, Rachel Bray (2009) has observed that women with HIV emphasized the need to maintain their extended family's reputation as well as their own positions within the family. She suggested: "The women's careful maintenance of kin relationships, often including periods of social and emotional distance, seemed to place them in the strongest position to claim familial support in the future" (2009, 176). In other words, by not drawing on kin ties, women attempted to circumvent negative sentiments that might arise because of their HIV diagnosis. Bray's insightful observations help explain how the appearance of a lack of illness management might actually be a desperate strategy to sustain familial ties and future resources not just for women but also for their children.

Parker Shipton's (2007) concept of entrustment is helpful for further disentangling the exchanges between Munyongo and Sarafina and their kin and, more broadly, understanding how familial commitments are worked out in an HIV era. Shipton uses the term entrustment to understand credit and debt in cultural-economic terms, which go beyond understandings of credit and debt in terms of formal institutions and arrangements. Entrustment is, in Shipton's terms, "an idea one step more abstract, and a shade more inclusive, than credit" (10). It "implies an obligation, but not necessarily an obligation to repay like with like, as a loan might imply. Whether an entrustment or transfer is returnable in kind or in radically different form—be it economic, political, symbolic, or some mixture of these—is a matter of cultural context and strategy" (11).

Entrustments include not just money and things, but also persons. Sending and receiving children of relatives is a form of entrustment and obligation. As I demonstrated in chapter 2, the exchange of children among kin has been the norm in Zambia, though the practice has changed in the context of HIV and AIDS. Munyongo's insistence on Sarafina's holiday visit was highly symbolic in terms of how she perceived herself repaying Sarafina for the care Sarafina had been giving her. It also enabled Munyongo and Sarafina to uphold their family responsibilities and relations to kin through sending Sarafina, while enabling Sarafina to receive some help under the guise of holiday.

Entrustments of a different sort—those more directly related to Munyongo's illness—might have shifted the balance of power, placing Sarafina and Munyongo in positions to repay relatives in the future or straining relations if future repayment was viewed as unlikely. As Shipton has argued, people who foster children in order to lessen the burden of care on a sending household "are doing a favor that puts them in a way on top (even at the risk of taking on a headache) and gives them advantage in future dealings. This leads to the issue of class" (2007, 31). This was a class issue that related also to how Sarafina was perceived and what effects that might have on the resources she received. Munyongo suggested that the future dealings that her sisters' children had with relatives were as orphans. The family resented the children's mother who had not only shirked her responsibilities but also brought TB into the family. Munyongo worked hard to avoid receiving blame and to circumvent such impressions of herself and Sarafina.

An entrustment approach helps us better understand the commitments that people make or attempt to avoid in illness. It also offers insight on how women and children experienced their commitments in ways that shaped illness management strategies. This is a matter of much concern in the context of HIV as development actors assess the state of families and care for the ill and children. Munyongo and Sarafina's case demonstrates what a number of scholars and activists have claimed: that previous assumptions about the extended family's ability to fill in the gaps of state care during crisis insufficiently address the inordinate stress placed on families within the HIV epidemic. Yet, Munyongo and Sarafina's case—as much as it shows need and stress—does not necessarily suggest household insularity or a breakdown in kinship. In fact, there were forms of exchange that were taking place, just not exchange related to Munyongo's illness, for better or worse. The extended family seemed intact at the end of my study, with few if any outward displays of resentment toward Munyongo. Avoidance appeared as an anticipatory strategy so that other, mostly future, needs could be fulfilled either in the case of Munyongo's death or her recovery.

Conclusion

Illness introduces many uncertainties, particularly in settings of privation, such as George. In this chapter, I have focused on the uncertainties women faced and the networks of support that women cultivated both with and through their children. There is a larger story within men's illness trajectories, which I have not covered. Nevertheless, in George, the social and material costs of becoming ill were more severe for women. This fact was evident in the differences between the types of kinship care received by sick men and women. Sick men received primary care from their wives, sisters, and mothers. Women, especially married, widowed, and divorced women with young children, received their care predominantly from their children. The stark differences in kinship care for men and women reflect the structural and social inequalities that shape women's responsibilities and access to resources.

If we are to understand how women manage and strategize their kinship obligations within the HIV epidemic, we must also consider what children accomplish for women. It is well documented that women take on the largest burdens of care work in households and families around the world. In the HIV epidemic, women's obligations to give care are expansive. Whether they are well or ill, women must prioritize the care they give. As I showed in this chapter, children could provide flexible care that women could not. Sarah's sister devised a way to help Sarah through sending her daughter to Sarah's house. Not only was she unavailable to help. Under the constraints placed on Sarah by her husband, no other relatives were welcome in Sarah's home and Sarah could not move out without disrupting her own marriage and identity in the process. At the same time, gendered obligations to help kin were felt at a young age, and Tracy expressed a strong sense of responsibility for Sarah's well-being.

A woman's illness created more than a crisis in care that children needed to fill. It created a disruption in the life course that carried implications for the future relationships and identities of women and the children in their care.[14] The experiences of Sarah and her sons and Munyongo and Sarafina demonstrate the difficult decisions women must make within the current contexts in order to guard their futures and the futures of their children. In Sarah's case, she expressed a need to remain married in order to protect herself and her children from destitution. To sustain her marriage and also sustain her children, she had to receive care from her children. However, not fulfilling her mothering duties also threatened her ties to her children and, thus, Sarah protected her identity as a mother. The flexible care that her niece Tracy offered became integral to Sarah's strategies. As Sarah herself described, Tracy became her mother. In the process, Tracy enabled Sarah to remain a mother to her children.

Munyongo and Sarafina's case offers yet another perspective in which the absence of kin involvement was, in fact, an aspect of illness management. Munyongo rejected the help of relatives who came to her house and avoided asking for help for Sarafina. In such rejection, there was much more at stake than care for Munyongo. Also at stake was Sarafina's present and future care. Munyongo and Sarafina's actions demonstrated the uncertainty that TB and other HIV-related illnesses bring in George. Munyongo aimed to safeguard her own and her daughter's life after her illness, when she would return to work and Sarafina to a better school. At the same time, she had to prepare her daughter for her death. Munyongo died in 2009, and Sarafina went to live with relatives outside of George. I do not know how effective their strategies were for managing Sarafina's future resources and identity because I have not been able to find Sarafina since she moved. Though there are many things I will not know, one thing remains clear: Munyongo and Sarafina's case compels us to recognize the varied ways in which adults and children prepare for uncertain futures and how this has become an impossible task within current conditions.

CHAPTER 6

Children and Global Health

Several months after Abby's mother was diagnosed with TB, Abby spoke the following words into my recorder: "When someone is sick in a family it affects everyone. They get worried. Some start thinking that the person might never recover or might die. Some worry because they don't have money to buy a coffin if she or he dies." Abby's close tying of sickness to death demonstrates the violence wrought by economic downturns and neoliberal projects, which have affected the state's capacity to mitigate such large-scale suffering and the capacities of families to care for the ill, in life and after death.

TB, other AIDS-related illnesses, malaria, malnutrition, substance abuse, and violence have severely reduced healthy life years in George. This reality was brought home to me every day when I walked through George Health Centre's entrance. And, in the past few years, a number of people who appeared throughout this book have died: Moffatt (Stephen's father), Munyongo (Sarafina's mother), Victor (Irene and Floyd's father), Musonda (Paul and Luka's father), Enelesi (Annie's mother).

Shared vulnerabilities accompany illness and death. Abby made these vulnerabilities evident as she continued her recording: "It would hurt me very badly if my mother had died when she was sick with TB." She quietly asked: "Who would take care of me? As to my side, I always pray to God to let my mother take care of me at least up to a stage where I can take care of myself and do the same for my sister and my brother. Not her dying, leaving me at this stage. No! No! Because some aunts say: 'They are orphans, I will do whatever I want to do with them.' That's what happens to orphans. They later become street kids." Abby connected her mother's possible death to her own social death, personalizing the representations of childhood created within the humanitarian response to HIV.

Yet Abby also punctuated her observations with optimism, saying: "Sometimes you might get very sick. Then people start saying that you are going to die, but surprisingly you recover, then gain weight even better than the way you were [before you became sick]." She concluded her recording with the words: "Life is wonderful. Everyone wants to live because life is wonderful." Abby's emphasis on recovery and life revealed emergent hope. She hinted at a newer aspect of the geography of infectious disease in Zambia and elsewhere—the growing presence of medical technologies that, at least in dominant ideology, sustain life and make a person even better than they were before they fell ill.

The second chances at life that TB and HIV treatment have offered some people in George are notable. Take for example Sarah, whose niece became her "mother,"[1] and Maureen, who asserted that her children provided most of her care, even though everyone expected it was the "elders."[2] During my fieldwork in 2007 and 2008, I witnessed both Sarah and Maureen as they recovered their health in ways that were unexpected, almost miraculous. When I visited in 2014, Sarah appeared in even better health than when I last saw her, and Maureen was so busy with work that we were not able to arrange a visit.

It is little wonder that issues of both living and dying preoccupied Abby and other children and shaped their caregiving strategies. In George, medications are available as they never have been before. At the same time, health services are severely strained, and individuals and families must go to great lengths to receive care for TB, HIV, and many other conditions. Throughout this book I have shown that, within such a context, children refashioned biomedical materials and knowledge, as well as child protection discourses and local understandings of children's roles, to fit their circumstances and needs. At the heart of understanding how they did so and what was at stake is the notion of care—both the care children gave and the care they attempted to receive.

A focus on children's caregiving offers an alternative heuristic for understanding dominant themes in global health and humanitarian work, such as familial caregiving for children and the sick, intergenerational communication about illness, the pharmaceuticalization of public health, universal treatment programs, and gender inequities in illness and care work, among others. In what follows, I reiterate the major lessons I have learned from working with children in George, and I offer new insights. Because I believe strongly that children's perspectives are needed for a fuller understanding of global health problems, I also outline approaches to include children in future global health studies and work.

REPRESENTING CHILDREN

One of the many challenges I faced in conducting research with children was how to consider children's perspectives in the context of a stigmatized, "adult" disease and in realms where their views have been traditionally excluded from

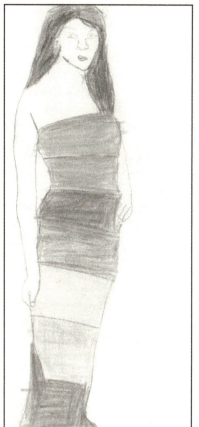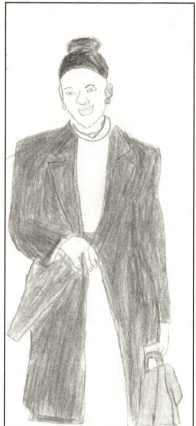

Figs. 6.1 and 6.2 Two of many drawings of women's fashion that Irene made for me. Drawings by Irene, age twelve.

anthropological analyses, such as in caregiving and therapy management.[3] It is not easy to learn from children in any setting, but it is particularly difficult within settings of adversity. The ethical issues I faced were many, as I have acknowledged throughout the book and most fully in my discussion of naming TB. As I was leaving Zambia to return to the United States in 2008, I was reminded that many ethical challenges remain in representing children's lives to a wider audience.[4]

In September of that year, I attended a Lusaka-based TB conference for practitioners who worked with the Consortium to Respond Effectively to the AIDS/ TB Epidemic, a multi-country effort. Since 2005, I had worked sporadically outside of George on TB-reduction programs implemented by researchers from the Zambia AIDS Related Tuberculosis Project. We were presenting our findings related to an intervention that included schoolchildren in TB reduction activities in a number of sites around Zambia.[5] The presentation included drawings that my colleagues and I had asked the schoolchildren to make during the final assessment stage of the project. In those drawings, the children depicted TB and HIV services in their communities.

My colleague, Virginia Bond, presented the materials, flipping through slides of children's drawings of clinics, TB Corners, and HIV testing services. She paused on a particular drawing to explain its significance. It was a particularly artful drawing, and I noticed many people smile when it appeared on the screen. The man seated next to me leaned over and whispered: "Now that one is going to be an architect." I might not have taken note of his comment had I not received a range of similar comments after the presentation about how good the drawings were. Such comments centered on children's skills and potential future professions, glossing over both the severity and importance of what the children were actually depicting. These are comments that I have received in other forums and are not particular to the people who participated in this meeting. Even I found myself awed by the skill with which twelve-year-old Irene executed her drawings of women's fashions (figs. 6.1 and 6.2).

In reality, the children participating in the schoolchild intervention, just as the children in my study, were unlikely to become architects and fashion designers because of where they were born. The ease with which we consider children's drawings in the future tense ignores this injustice. Aesthetics can be distracting, eliding a political and economic analysis of the worlds in which children live. The comments betrayed something equally as insidious. It is impossible to take children's knowledge and experiences seriously when they are viewed as becoming rather than being. If we only look at children's drawings with a view of the future, we cannot take seriously the challenges and hurts they face as children in the present, and we cannot take seriously what they anticipate for their own futures.

Beyond Children-as-Victims: Toward an Understanding of Children's Health Agency

There is no denying that children living in heavily TB- and HIV-affected areas are, in many senses of the word, victims of global processes that have sustained inequalities in health and resources. At the risk of sounding repetitive, I describe again the many factors that have negatively affected the children in my study and were clearly out of the children's control. Well before the children were born, a declining economy, neoliberal policies and structural adjustment programs, increased urban poverty, a gutted healthcare system, the emergence of HIV, among other factors, created conditions ripe for a sustained TB epidemic. International policies in the 1990s led to a shortage of TB treatment in Zambia as well as the inaccessibility of ARVs (for HIV) for most citizens until 2004, even as ART had been available to many people living in wealthy countries for years. Policies and funding streams have changed, and there are glimmers of hope, but the roll out of ART and the greater availability of TB medications alone have not ended suffering, especially for the most marginalized.

Viewing children as victims of these processes, however, is overly simplistic. It casts children as passive and dismisses their points of view. Even though the children in my study were not alive during the 1980s or most of the 1990s, the changes that occurred during these years were etched into the social memory. It is impossible to overstate the importance of medicine in a context where people were left to die or the meaning of a TB or HIV diagnosis for families that have said goodbye to too many relatives. This history is part of children's communication about illness, the ways in which they involved themselves in care for themselves and their sick guardians, and their approaches to biomedicine, schooling, and much more.

I have shown throughout this book that children did not see themselves as passive, even within the most challenging contexts. Abby was one of the children who attended my first children's workshop, which focused on children's understandings of and contributions to health in George. Olivious, Emily, and I had practiced what we would say at the workshop, repeatedly. We wanted the children to know that we had organized the workshops specifically for the children to share their views, and that we did not intend to teach the children. As Olivious explained our purpose, the children sat stoically, hanging onto her words, but with few visible responses to what she was saying. Then she finally said: "In this workshop, you are the teachers. Today, we are learning from you." Abby jumped up, gasped loudly. With her hand over her mouth, she grinned widely. The rest of the children paused, smiled, and looked at one another.

Even this well-rehearsed, conscious effort to listen to children was challenging. Prior to the workshops, Emily expressed to me that she was anxious about the answers the children might come up with and how we should respond to them. To her, it made no sense to let the sessions play out with very little adult input. Emily is a counselor and wonderful teacher to her own children, nieces, nephews, and grandchildren. She held a keen awareness of the inequalities in access to knowledge the children faced. When the children started to give what in fact were wrong answers, I felt the same anxiety as Emily. Should I explain that ARVs were not a disease, as expressed by some children? What if the children learned incorrect information from my workshops and used what they learned to inform their understandings of illness and their interactions in their families? And what if they spread what they learned to their teachers, parents, and guardians, who would view me as giving misinformation or, alternatively, use what the children said to inform their own views? My acknowledged concern that the children would see me as a teacher obscured my own rather subconscious understanding of myself as a knowledge producer. In the end, we thanked the children for participating in the workshops and told them how much we had learned from them. We framed the conclusion to emphasize the biomedically accurate information given to us by the children and downplayed answers that did not fit into our belief system.

What is important is the contradiction between how social science researchers may view adults' responses and children's responses differently and what this obscures in our analyses. For example, I at times heard adults say that HIV or AIDS comes from or is produced by TB. This, to me, was an astute observation that, in few words, tells us that HIV status was often unknown until a person faces a crisis illness such as TB. It also revealed the unidirectional flow of TB patients into HIV counseling and testing services and the close social and biomedical connections between TB and HIV. In other words, I did not see this phrase as particularly inaccurate according to biomedical understandings of HIV and TB, even though it was technically incorrect. In contrast, when children told me that ARV was a disease or that ARVs cured TB, I immediately wanted to correct them and I viewed the children as misinformed. A closer analysis of children's accounts of ARVs as disease, however, reveals many important things about the ways in which children learned about disease through medicine. It reveals one of many ways in which people in George maintained sociality and expressed care for one another through invoking medication rather than diagnosis. So often, as adults, we feel the need to teach children and prepare them for the future. We forget just how much they have to offer us in the present.

To view children as agents is to give credit where credit has long been due for children's in-depth knowledge of their social worlds, and also for their actions in shaping those worlds. Children, as I have shown throughout this book, do many things that we are not paying attention to because we do not expect or want children to do them and because our methodologies for viewing such problems exclude children. The frequency with which the children in my study ensured that adults received and took their TB medications is one case in point.

Yet, we must be careful how we envision children as health agents. In much public health work, children have been recruited to share information and encourage particular health behaviors. This, in my opinion, is not honoring children's agency. It is seeing them as megaphones to disseminate messages more widely than public health actors can typically reach. Such a view exemplifies an adult or elitist perspective—the intentions of children who participate in such interventions are left unexamined because they are expected to align with those of public health actors.[6]

To view children as health agents is to honor children's everyday efforts to maintain dignity and sustain lives within exceptionally difficult circumstances. This means seeing them as part of the social basis of health and exploring the entanglements of the social and biomedical as experienced, enacted, and lived by children.[7] This is not to argue that we privilege children's actions and perspectives within illness.[8] It is to suggest the necessity of viewing children as people who act within social contexts and in relation to and relationship with other people in their families and communities.

Beyond Children-as-Victims: Toward an Understanding of Adults' Health Agency

A move toward understanding children's health agency holds potential to open up new interpretations of the health agency of adults. Dominant discourses about HIV, TB, and other infectious diseases frequently focus on children as the innocent victims of the risky behaviors of adults: babies exposed to HIV through mother-to-child transmission, children orphaned when parents die of HIV-related infections, and children exposed to abuse and labor (Fassin 2013). This framing of children as passive victims of adult actions is related to the preoccupation with individual (adult) behavior change that has dominated global public health responses to infectious disease.[9] When paired with the notion of children as victims vis-à-vis adult behavior, it not only exaggerates adult agency but also exacerbates the blaming of adults for children's circumstances, especially adults who fail to alter their behaviors in specific ways.

My discussion of disclosure to children offers an example of the necessity of a relational view of children's and adults' health agency. In recent years, public health practitioners and researchers have identified nondisclosure of HIV status to children as a behavior that adults might change to the benefit of their children and themselves. This suggestion holds many assumptions, two of which I cover below: first, that adult talk is unconstrained; and, second, that adults possess the power to give children agency or take it away. Both assumptions are problematic—the first because it exaggerates adults' agency and ignores the histories and lived experiences that have shaped such concealments and the second because it simultaneously denies children health agency and exaggerates their agency.

First, issues of power and social position shape what is said, who does the talking, and what remains unsaid. This clearly puts children at a structural disadvantage in terms of speaking and being told about HIV and TB. However, this does not mean that adult talk is unconstrained. As the guardians in my study showed, there were many constraints on their talk related to the extreme and uncertain conditions in which they lived and their desires to nurture their children within such conditions. Much work on disclosure of parental HIV to children has not adequately addressed these constraints. A lack of direct naming is often framed as cultural, with silence equated with cultural differences in talk about sex and death with children. While identifying that adults face challenges in speaking about HIV, such an analysis of silence as cultural overlooks the historical, economic, and social factors that have compelled concealment. It conflates structural violence and cultural difference.[10]

Second, in the commentaries on disease disclosure, silence and disclosure are positioned in opposition, with silence implying passivity and a lack of communication and disclosure standing for action and communication. However, instead of being passively unaware, children held detailed knowledge of TB in the absence of a named disease. Children actively collected knowledge of disease through attention to small signs on their sick relatives' bodies and changes in their houses and households. Children, too, engaged in strategic concealments to show care to the sick. Their awareness and actions complicate the dichotomous thinking embedded in the research on disclosure, which has led to claims that adult disclosure will shift children from passive victims of HIV to active participants in shaping their own care and that of their family members. As I have shown, belief in this trajectory ignores the amount of care and communication accomplished in the absence of a named disease and also exaggerates children's abilities to change their situations when disease is named.

My analysis of disclosure raises a further point about adult behavior change interventions aimed at children's well-being. The conceptualization of disclosure as beneficial to children is grounded in a not-so-subtle assumption that outsiders know what type of communication is best for children. This is a privileged gaze that allows a willful ignorance of other forms of communication. I have suggested a different starting point, which identifies that communication and action can take many forms that may not be readily obvious to outsiders. This starting point allows us to investigate a range of other important issues, such as how people approach intergenerational care, maintain relationships, and attempt to secure resources within tremendous constraint. Investigating these aspects brings us closer to answering the bigger question that underpins almost all research and commentaries on disclosure to children, which is: How might the needs of sick adults and their young children be met to permit their continued relationships with one another?

What We Miss When We Miss Children

Many globally produced policies and programs explicitly target children. There are many others that target adults and overlook children almost entirely. Until 2013, when the World Health Organization declared childhood TB as one of its priority areas, children were rarely commented on in debates and discussion about TB treatment. And even still, the emphasis on childhood TB has not been on understanding children's experiences and social worlds, but on developing and providing technologies—diagnostic tools and specialized child-friendly TB treatment formulas. For this reason, I ask: What do we miss when we overlook children's experiences, actions, and perspectives?

Throughout this book, I have offered many reasons for why we cannot dismiss children. I reinforce these reasons with yet another example, journalist David Baron's (2010) account of healthcare rationing in Zambia, which was part of a Public Radio International series on healthcare rationing across four countries—South Africa, England, India, and Zambia. In Baron's report, he suggested that, in Zambia, healthcare is unintentionally rationed by implicit factors. The implicit factor he described in his report was the long queues at ARV clinics since the roll-out of no-cost treatment. This "rationing by queue" is of course no revelation to Zambians, who will readily divulge and complain about how long they have to wait to receive public healthcare. Baron went on to suggest that a variety of factors determined whether or not a person could wait. As he suggested: "This kind of implicit rationing may discourage certain categories of patients—for instance, those with young children or with full-time jobs."

As biomedical technologies to treat TB and manage HIV become increasingly available around the world and as pharmaceuticals become a main form of public health delivery, there has been an increasing recognition that relationships affect treatment seeking. Community support is now recognized as integral to the implementation of DOTS protocol, and a number of NGOs have assisted the government health centers in Zambia to make community DOT possible. But these programs of patient support come and go in George, with the ebb and flow of international funding. The TB treatment supporters I have known through the years are dedicated, but they are overworked and their work is frequently unremunerated. In other words, despite these efforts and changes, treatment adherence continues to be made possible (or not) through familial relationships. A series of social and economic differences structure the ways in which particular individuals are able to wait for medications and others are not, with age- and gender-related effects. Women carry out much work of collecting medicine, especially medicine for men. Other people, mostly women and children, make waiting in queues possible by providing childcare or household work.

The children I knew in George were integral to TB treatment adherence. They carried out household chores, sibling care, and care for the sick that made the collection of medication possible, raising questions about how children figure into such as system of healthcare rationing. Beyond medicine collection, the children expounded on the rules of treatment and reminded adults to take their medications. They knew where medicines were stored and when they needed to be taken. The reality that children were doing something to make treatment accessible and adherence possible is worthy of acknowledgment. While TB treatment is available, this does not mean that it is accessible. The institutional and medical infrastructure to ensure access is much better than it was in the past, but it is still severely lacking. Children help make up for the absences. It may not be an exaggeration to say that the efforts of children to keep people on treatment optimally benefit the state and beyond.

TB treatment is a resource for children at a time when resources are especially scarce. As I have shown, there were so many things about TB that excluded children. Children were not often welcomed in TB Corners. They were sometimes moved out of households as families attempted to accommodate the needs of patients and avoid transmission to children. In most households I worked in, adults expressed a very real concern about spreading TB to their children. Clinical advice to avoid transmission and received wisdom, passed down from more stringent clinical rules in the previous decades, took away some things that affirmed children's relationships with their guardians, such as eating together and sleeping close. In such a context, the availability of pharmaceuticals and the ideals about patient support became vital resources for children, even though neither was intended for them. As I have shown, children repurposed these materials and rules, offering their own forms of patient support. In the process, they enacted claims to particular people and households and worked to transform their relationships and retain normative identities. There was much at stake, including the biological life of a beloved relative and the social life and future of the child.

Remaining Close

As my research in the households drew to a close, I worried about the effects of an abrupt departure on some of the children with whom I was especially close. I carried out a number of activities to thank them for spending time with me. The last set of children's workshops that I held celebrated children's participation in the study. I expressed my gratitude through words and small gifts. And on my final visits to each household, I gave cards to the households, with enclosed pieces of paper that described some of my research findings. I did not wish to be the researcher who collected her data and never returned, though life circumstances have led me closer to these fears than I feel comfortable admitting. My soonest return would not be until 2014.

Back in 2008, on what I assumed would be my final visit to Irene's household, I gave Irene and her brother a stack of paper. They had drawn through reams during the year I had been visiting them and, while I knew I should look beyond the aesthetic appeal of their drawings, I still assumed that they enjoyed drawing as a personal endeavor. Two weeks later, I passed by their home unexpectedly to give them some books I had received from a friend as a donation to the children in my study. Irene was clearly surprised to see me, saying: "I didn't draw anything for you because I didn't think you were coming back." At that moment, only after the research had ended, I realized that her drawings served as a means to cultivate a relationship with me, to be closer to me than she might have been without the drawings.

If we do not question the ways in which children engage us as researchers, we will never fully comprehend what they are telling and showing us. In my research, children's uses of my methods fit within their overall strategies to sustain relationships. The drawings children gave me as gifts and drew as assignments induced me to return to their homes and strengthened our connections to one another. Even if they were skeptical of the topics I suggested, most children completed the assignments, demonstrating that help is what nurtures relationships. It is with this understanding that I view Abby's final drawing to Olivious and me with mixed feelings. The drawing was of colorful flowers, hearts, and curvy designs; the word "love" embedded into the shapes. At the top of the page, she wrote in large letters "I Love You Olivia and Jean." In smaller lettering on the bottom she wrote, "This is love for you."

The love Abby offered to Olivious and me reminds me that we, too, became enmeshed in social relations of care, if only for a brief moment in time. Expressing love was how the children held onto relationships that mattered, when they were at their most fragile. Putting love into words sustained relationships and compelled people to be closer to each other, both physically and emotionally. When attempts to maintain physical proximity failed, expressions of love became attempts to retain closeness, to remember people once they were gone.[11] I am reminded of eleven-year-old Eliya, who addressed his father, as he whispered softly into my recorder, "Father, don't worry. I will take care of my mother and always love you. I will never forget you because I know you are happy, wherever you are. You were very kind. May you rest in peace."

Childhood Tuberculosis

I returned to George Health Centre in June 2014, after a six-year absence. When I left in 2008, the TB Corner was in transition, moving out of the open-air carport, a space it had occupied temporarily each day for several years. At that time, an international NGO was building a new, permanent TB Corner, on an open plot of land, close to the entrance of the Health Centre but tucked away from the daily hubbub of clinic activities. By 2014, this new TB Corner had been in use for years. I arrived to see it for the first time late on a Monday afternoon, well after the daily drug distribution had finished. I walked, together with Olivious, through its open doors and into the large room where patients and their family members sat each day while waiting to receive their medication. This room took up most of the space in the building, and there were two smaller offices used by staff, visiting researchers, and for more private conversations.

For just a moment, Olivious and I were the only people in the room. We stood together, feeling a cross breeze blow through windows. The permanence of the concrete walls struck me. TB had a location. The TB nurses and TB treatment supporters no longer had to haul paper charts, medicine bottles, benches, and tables out of storage each morning and into storage each afternoon. They had not done so in years. Sleek educational posters hung on the walls, alongside carefully handwritten signs that offered instructions to staff, volunteers, and patients. Files were arranged on wooden shelves that hung on the wall next to the table where the TB nurse sat as she called up each patient.

The blue plastic cover on the nurse's table caught my eye. It read ZAMINDS—referring to the Association of Medical Doctors of Asia—Multisectoral and Integrated Development Services, an organization funded by the Japanese government that has carried out many TB projects with George Health Centre. I looked at the Zambian Government and ZAMINDS logos that were printed across the cloth and was reminded of how public-private partnerships and multilateral funding shaped the Health Centre's ability to treat the many people suffering from TB. Then I noticed something about the patients treated through this particular project. They were children. Not only did TB have a permanent location in the clinic; children had a place in this location.

In October 2013, the World Health Organization released its first ever roadmap for the prevention of childhood TB. This marked a substantial shift from the adult-centricity of most medical and public health programs on TB. The roadmap—a thirty-eight-page report that offered guidance and resources—called childhood TB a missed opportunity:

> Many children who present with TB disease represent an opportunity missed by the health system to have prevented the disease. This is particularly the case for infants and young children: studies consistently show that most cases of TB in children occur in those with a known contact who has been diagnosed with TB, which is frequently a parent or another close relative of the child. Infants and young children are at particularly high risk for severe, disseminated TB disease and for TB-related mortality. And yet it is all too common to have the child of a parent who has TB to present with TB meningitis, which is frequently fatal, and if not, often results in marked and permanent disability. This could be prevented by screening children who are contacts of people diagnosed with TB and by providing preventive therapy for children younger than five years of age at the time TB is diagnosed in a parent or family member. (World Health Organization 2013, 11)

In certain ways, this focus on missed healthcare opportunities was responding to the pleas I heard from guardians in George, who expressed concerns over what would happen if their children became sick with the disease. The guardians wanted the clinic to do more to help prevent TB transmission to their children. The WHO's focus also responded, very belatedly, to a study conducted in Zambia from 1997 to 2000, in which researchers at the University Teaching Hospital carried out autopsies of children who had died with respiratory disease. These autopsies showed a high rate of undiagnosed TB disease in the children (Chintu et al. 2002). Another article, published just prior to the release of the WHO's *Roadmap for Childhood Tuberculosis*, reasserted the need for better prevention of childhood TB in Zambia and also better diagnostic and treatment services for children with active disease (Kapata et al. 2013).

Floyd Makeka, a lead TB treatment supporter whom I have known for years, came out of the TB Corner's back office. My unfamiliar presence in the space seemed to make him, too, see the many changes that had occurred through the years. The three of us walked around the room. We chatted about our health and our families. Olivious had married, had a son, and moved away from George since the last time she and Mr. Makeka met. Mr. Makeka's children were small when I knew him. They were grown now. His wife continued to have back problems but was, generally, in good health. With the help of their children, she had started a new business selling grilled fish and meat in the evenings. Mr. Makeka was busier than ever at the TB Corner. Still, the household struggled to make ends meet. TB treatment supporters such as Mr. Makeka are considered volunteers, receiving small stipends, or no stipends at all, for work that requires tremendous amounts of time as well as physical and emotional energy, and also carries risks.[1]

Mr. Makeka took me into the office to introduce me to the new TB nurse, Mercy Mwale. Ms. Mwale, it seemed, brought energy to the Corner that matched the hope radiating from its walls. Upon learning about my previous work with the children, she grew serious. They were struggling to serve children who had TB, she said. According to their records, there were thirty-eight children (from newborns up to sixteen years old) with active TB that needed treatment from the Corner. Twenty-four more children were on isoniazid preventive therapy to treat latent, or inactive, TB infections.

One year prior to my visit, and with the help of ZAMINDS, the TB Corner established Friday as the designated day to treat children. While the pediatric TB day and extra supportive services that the project provided had benefits, the project was coming to an end, and it had exposed the complexities of social issues involved in treatment. Not all children's guardians collected the children's medicines regularly, and the clinic workers struggled to get guardians to return. The Friday schedule offered one way of focusing just on children's special needs. It seemed like this was a good thing in their opinion, but it also represented a burden when adult household members were also on treatment and needed to come to the clinic on other days to collect their medication. Older children sometimes came alone, and these children seemed to do okay, at least with collecting the medication. The entire process of scaling up services to children revealed even further what both Ms. Mwale and Mr. Makeka already knew: a range of social and economic factors structure who gets treatment and who does not in resource-poor settings.

The international focus on childhood TB has created new types of TB patients—children. The international scramble to diagnose and treat children with TB is vital. However, child-specific diagnostics and treatments, alone, will not solve the problem. Without adequate institutional and economic resources, children and their family members will continue to do much of the work of supporting treatment, this time for children. Children's chances on TB treatment, just as the chances of the sick adults whom I wrote about throughout this book, will depend on the contingencies of their relationships.

The new focus on children raises many questions: For example, what will it mean to be a child, or family member of a child, diagnosed with TB, a disease with a long and complicated history? How will TB diagnosis reflect on a child's personhood and life prospects and on the personhood and life prospects of other family members, particularly family members who have suffered from the disease? How will treatment shape the interdependence between children and specific adults? What types of work are children doing to support their own treatment and the treatment of siblings? What are the implications for women's livelihoods and security? Who will receive blame if treatment fails?

Answering these questions will be critical to determining the directions that TB programs need to take and the institutional supports needed to assist children and their families. The answers are not found in boardrooms of international organizations or in large-scale epidemiological studies. They rest heavily on an understanding of the forms that care takes in particular settings and how these forms transcend the boundaries of home, clinic, and nation, and change through time. Such answers, as I have argued throughout this book, demand an ethnographic approach to illness that underscores children's actions, relationships, dependencies, and interdependencies.

Notes

INTRODUCTION

1. In Zambia, the number of new cases of TB during the year 2014 was estimated at 406 in every 100,000 people, indicating one of the highest burdens of TB in the world (World Health Organization 2015a).

2. These figures do not account for latent infections. Latent TB infections are asymptomatic. Such infections do not make a person sick nor are they infectious. It is estimated that 2 billion people around the world carry such infections. The risk of latent infection progressing to active infection is higher when people have comorbidities or face other stressors that affect their immune systems, such as displacement, homelessness, and chronic hunger.

3. See also Paul Farmer on this point. He identifies that disparities in wealth and health "remind us of links, rather than disjunctures, between settings of affluence and privation" (2013, xv).

4. See Farmer (1997) and Erin Koch (2013) for their arguments about the political economic structuring of the TB epidemic. Both argue against a view that TB and other infectious diseases are the result of individual behaviors and, thus, preventable primarily through behavior change interventions.

5. In 2014, around 13.3 percent of Zambian adults (ages fifteen to forty-nine) were estimated to have HIV (UNAIDS 2014). Demonstrating the synergy between HIV and TB, more than 62 percent of people diagnosed with TB also test positive for HIV (WHO 2015a).

6. I borrow the phrase "ugly death" from Livingston (2012) because it is such an apt term for describing the terrible bodily and social devastation that deaths due to TB-HIV have caused.

7. Maureen's diagnosis of HIV before TB was not typical. During the years of my research, most people I knew received a TB diagnosis first and then an HIV diagnosis.

8. See Luke Messac and Krishna Prabhu's (2013) excellent analysis and description of the political economic changes that transformed global health approaches from prevention to treatment, specifically for HIV and AIDS.

9. Susan Reynolds Whyte and her coauthors (2014b) have used the idea of second chances to explore the meaning of ART, and the reprieve it offered from death, for the first generation of people who had access to ART in Uganda.

10. See Ruth Evans and Saul Becker (2009). In a different example, the United Kingdom (Office for National Statistics 2013) collects data on children's unpaid carework for family members, friends, and neighbors. The 2011 census identified 117,918 children (ages five to seventeen years old) as providers of unpaid care.

11. In Zambia, 1.4 million children aged seventeen and under have experienced the death of at least one biological parent due to any cause (UNICEF 2016).

12. See Fiona Ross (2010), who has argued that models of disease that view illness as outside of everyday life do not fit certain settings where illness is the norm, rather than the exception.

13. For example, the Global Fund partnership (2016) alone allocates nearly 4 billion dollars each year toward HIV, TB, and malaria programs.

14. See Cole and Durham's (2007) edited volume on how global restructuring shapes and is affected by intimate aspects of daily life. The volume focuses on the importance of analyzing relationships between age categories, rather than focusing on one singular category in isolation.

15. This statistic comes from the World Health Organization's (2013) roadmap for ending childhood TB. However, the authors recognize that this percentage is problematic because children in high burden areas can account for as much as 10 to 20 percent of the TB burden. Further, diagnosing TB in children is highly difficult and there is likely a much higher burden than currently recognized.

16. See chapter 3 for why I did not directly refer to a parent or guardian's illness as TB.

17. See Bluebond-Langner (1978), Hardman (1973), Schwartzman (1978).

18. For example, in *Key Concepts in Childhood Studies*, Allison James and Adrian James (2012), two preeminent researchers in childhood studies, categorize children's care under the heading of "Work and Working Children."

19. For some examples, see Pamela Reynolds's (1991) research in Zimbabwe and Karen Tranberg Hansen's (1990) research in Zambia. See also Nicola Ansell and Lorraine van Blerk's (2004) article, which covers, among other topics, children's household work as a coping strategy within the HIV epidemic in Lesotho and Malawi.

20. Historian Philippe Ariès (1962) is often credited for the argument that childhood was not a fixed life stage. He provocatively suggested that, before the modern period, children were considered miniature adults who were immersed in the world of work, rather than separated from it. While his book was the subject of much scholarly debate, a central tenet of his argument—that childhood is a social construction—has shaped understandings of the cross-cultural variability in expectations and capacities of children to work.

21. Marjory Faulstich Orellana (2009) has argued for acknowledging the complexity of immigrant children and youth's translation work in the United States, including their language and culture brokering in doctors' offices and other health encounters, which is a form of care work.

22. This follows Angela Garcia's (2010) analysis of commensurability and care in the context of heroin addiction in New Mexico.

23. An emphasis on children's participation is part of a larger focus on children's right to participate in their communities, which has been written into the United Nations Convention on the Rights of the Child.

24. The Zambia AIDS Related Tuberculosis project is an organization that represents a longstanding affiliation between the University of Zambia and the London School of Hygiene and Tropical Medicine. This particular schoolchild project was funded by a grant from the Bill and Melinda Gates Foundation and was part of a larger multiyear study, the Zambia and South Africa Tuberculosis and AIDS Reduction Study (ZAMSTAR).

25. See an article I published with colleagues on the schoolchild intervention (Bond et al. 2010).

26. See some examples of this research in Zambia (Kaona et al. 2004; Mulenga et al. 2010; Mweemba et al. 2008).

27. Ian Harper's (2006) observations in Nepal and Koch's (2006, 2013) observations in Georgia both offer strong arguments for the use of ethnographic field methods to inform policies on TB treatment.

28. In *Writing Ethnographic Fieldnotes*, the authors refer to ethnographic fieldwork as a practice of "getting close." In their words, ethnographic research "minimally requires physical and social proximity to the daily rounds of people's lives and activities" (Emerson et al. 1995, 1–2).

29. My research affiliation with ZAMBART started in 2005. This affiliation carried many benefits. Outside of George, I was able to observe and participate in ZAMBART's TB control efforts and studies. In George, I shared space and camaraderie with the ZAMBART staff who worked at George Health Centre (chapter 4). While we shared space, we avoided recruiting the same households into our studies.

30. I was not able to visit all twenty-five households in 2014 because some people had moved outside of George or members had died and the households had dispersed.

31. The idea of comparison households extends from what public health practitioners call a case-control study, a method developed during the twentieth century as a time-efficient and low-cost method of studying chronic and emerging diseases, particularly in low-income countries. Generally speaking, the driving motivation behind such a model is the belief that in order to understand the effects of the presence of disease, we must also study its absence (Henneken and Buring 1987). In George, the distinctions between households with and without TB are artificial and time specific. Participants in most comparison households had cared for sufferers in the past and were caring for non-household TB sufferers in the present. Six months into the study, a woman living in one of the eight comparison households was diagnosed with TB.

32. I administered this 200 household survey to help me better understand what was unique to the 25 households and what was more widely shared by other households in George. More details on sampling strategy, variables, and analysis can be found in Hunleth et al. (2015).

33. See for example Gallacher and Gallagher (2008) and Hunleth (2011) for reflections on and critiques of the privileging of participatory research methods in childhood research.

34. Because the risk of TB transmission is greatest prior to treatment, we were the most cautious during the beginning of the research and at times when other people in the households showed signs of undiagnosed TB. There were several households, including in my comparison sample, where people became sick with TB after the start of the study.

35. See Hunleth (2011) for how such crises shape research with children.

36. This is a perspective expressed in recent work by anthropologists of global health (Adams et al. 2014; Pigg 2013).

37. Among these translation challenges was the translation from Nyanja and Bemba to English. Except where indicated, all of my conversations occurred in one of two Bantu languages, Nyanja or Bemba, with Emily and Olivious translating the words and meanings of what people were saying when I did not fully understand. Olivious transcribed all recorded conversations and interviews, and we discussed the transcripts and translations together. In the quotations in this book, I have worked to best preserve the meaning of what people were saying while keeping the wording understandable. In certain places I have used Nyanja words, with translations provided.

Chapter 1 — Growing Up in George

1. At the time that Luka made his drawing, Zambia had nine provinces. In 2011, President Sata declared a tenth province, Muchinga Province.

2. See Chawla (2002) and Young (2003) for how children understand and alter space created for and by adults.

3. A peri-urban area is defined by its existence on the outskirts of cities. It is an area between rural and urban, and most often marked by poverty, overcrowding, and an absence of sufficient amenities.

4. The settlement has gone by several names since Zambia's independence, though George is the one that remains consistently used today. Notably, the area was called Kapwepwe after Simon Kapwepwe, who fought for independence alongside Zambia's first president, Kenneth Kaunda. He served as the second vice president of Zambia until he and Kaunda developed differences and Kapwepwe established his own party.

5. By 1967, the population of George was quickly growing and estimated around 11,000 (Schlyter and Schlyter 1979).

6. Karen Tranberg Hansen (1997) offers an extensive account of the problems that occurred during upgrading.

7. See Biehl and Petryna (2013b) and Farmer et al. (2013) for more detailed accounts and histories of this shifting global health environment.

8. I was given this number by a community worker who worked in George Health Centre and with nongovernmental organizations in the settlement. An approximate number of 120,000 residents was displayed on a piece of poster paper that was taped on the wall in the dining area of George Health Centre.

9. See Hansen (1997) and Schlyter and Schlyter (1979) for extended discussions of the history and uses of the terms compound and mayadi in urban Zambia.

10. See also Swart-Kruger (2002), who has made similar observations in a squatter camp in South Africa.

11. For the first drawings, I asked the children to draw whatever they wanted, with no guidance or direction. After this first drawing, I offered topics for the children to base their drawings on.

12. Many people in George do not have electricity. Sixty-two out of 200 houses I surveyed were wired for electricity, though not all of these households had working electricity. Still, everyone in George is affected by outages in some way.

13. Without data from the past, it is even more difficult to discern whether water-drawing practices have changed because of the kajima setup. In the sample of 313 children ages six to fourteen years old from the 200 households I surveyed in George, respondents

reported that 54 percent of girls and 60 percent of boys between the ages of six and fourteen had not drawn water for their household in the past month. Most surveyed householders said that children between six and eight years old never drew water and those between nine and eleven only rarely did. When children between twelve and fourteen years old drew water, they only did so an average of once per week. These numbers seem quite low based on my observations of and conversations with children.

14. This average comes from my survey of 200 households in George.

15. Victim Support Units (VSUs) were integrated into police stations in Zambia during the late 1990s to address gender-related violence and rights issues. The VSUs focus on issues women and girls face such as property grabbing, abuse, and rape. Yet the benefits of reporting husbands and family members to the VSU was the subject of heated discussions among women in George, who worried that the fines and bribes demanded by the VSUs would take the last bits of money they and their families had, leaving them in a worse situation.

16. The children enjoyed having pictures to "talk with" when they used my tape recorder, so I used a book of international development drawings entitled *Where There is No Artist* (Rohr-Rouendaal 1997) to provide them with drawings on themes such as family, school, medicine, and illness.

17. The literacy rate, according to the *Millennium Development Goals Status Report 2005* (Ministry of Education 2006), progressively worsened for young people aged fifteen to twenty-four from 79 percent in 1990 to 70 percent in 2004. The decline in girls' literacy was even worse, falling from 75 percent in 1990 to 66 percent in 2004.

18. See, for example, a paper I published with colleagues (Bond et al. 2010) for a description of a schoolchild TB reduction program in Zambia. See also examples of child participatory programs initiated in other countries (Guang-Han et al. 2005; Onyango-Ouma et al. 2005) and a review of the literature on children's participation in disaster risk reduction activities (Muzenda-Mudavanhu 2016).

19. I have observed educational programs on both TB and HIV in schools in George. But the lessons I observed were clinical, didactic, and taught by individuals who lacked the resources to address such complex topics with children. The lessons seemed disconnected from children's experiences with illness in their everyday lives

CHAPTER 2 — RESIDENCE AND RELATIONSHIPS

1. A long literature in sub-Saharan Africa has identified the importance of child fostering or the entrustment of children to extended family members, for at least part of their childhoods, as a means of securing children's needs as well as dispersing the needs of households and extended families. This literature has identified children's exchange as a means of tying households and relatives together in the present as well as in the longer term. See Colson (1958) for examples from Zambia. Also see Shipton (2007) for examples from Kenya.

2. These answers were given to me during group discussions that took place in the children's workshops in June and July 2008.

3. This point resonates with Pamela Reynolds's (1991) characterization of children's agricultural labor in the lower Zambezi as flexible labor.

4. The children made this point clear in role plays they enacted on the topic of "being a child in a house."

5. See, for example, Klaits (2010) on the domestication of inequality in Botswana, in which he focuses on how women experience inequality in their domestic relationships and also how they attempt to bring this inequality under control.

6. See, for example, Fortes (1969) and Whyte et al. (2014).

7. See Shipton (2007) for a more recent account of giving and receiving children as a form of entrustment between kin.

8. For example, see Ansell and van Blerk (2004) on the balancing of needs in households through sending and receiving children.

9. For example, see UNICEF (2004) on the narrowing of extended family care, a term the report uses to characterize the limited availability of caregivers for children in need.

10. See Shipton (2007) on the class differences in child entrustment in Kenya. In Zambia, children's circulation has long been associated with differential abilities to support or educate a child, with children moving in to financially better off households or households better able to educate a child because of their resources or proximity to a school (Colson 1971; Hansen 1990; Lancaster 1981).

11. See Crehan (1997) on the flexibility of kinship descent rules.

12. This does not mean that the children were living with mothers and/or fathers or that all of the household members remained the same through time. For example, a child who was born into a household composed of her mother and maternal grandparents, but whose mother had moved away, was considered to have always lived with the household. This number also represents children who may have moved around George or to George, but whose moves were made as part of a household move, rather than the child's unaccompanied move into a new household.

13. Gonzalez de la Rocha (2007) describes that "myth of survival," suggesting that optimistic messages about the resourcefulness of the poor may not match reality or the impact of changing economies on poor people's lives.

14. See Archambault (2010), who describes how the growth of schooling and Christianity, among other changes, have placed pressure on the Maasai in Kenya to "modernize" family life.

15. See Whyte et al. (2014, 106) for similar assessment of ideals of kin responsibility in general in the HIV era.

16. Children moved in "just because" the child or someone in the household wanted to live together (n = 5).

17. I distinguish between Abby's uncle and Abby's mother's brother because, in the former, uncle served as a classificatory term. I am unsure how the man was related, except through Abby's mother.

18. I thank Musonda Simwinga for helping me with this point.

19. Similar to the view of children taken by adults in other parts of sub-Saharan Africa, children in George saw themselves as "potential" persons, "possessing limited competencies that gradually increase throughout the life cycle, with the ultimate goal of achieving full personhood" (Cheney 2007, 59).

20. Definitions of orphans have varied over the years, but a main definition used in global humanitarian work is a child who has lost either one or both parents.

21. I borrow this phrase from Meintjes and Geise (2006). Crivello and Chuta (2012) refer to orphans as the embodiment of child vulnerability. See also Ansell (2016) for an

examination of why Western observers have focused so heavily on orphans within the HIV crisis in sub-Saharan Africa.

22. The importance of children's holiday movements has been noted in passing by a number of social scientists in sub-Saharan, including Notermans (2008) and Ungruhe (2010).

23. See Hunleth et al. (2015) for an extended analysis of my quantitative survey on children's holidays.

24. See Reynolds (1991).

25. See Ansell (2016), Crivello and Chuta (2012), and Meintjes and Geise (2006). To address funding gaps, the category has been broadened to orphans and vulnerable children, or OVC. Still, orphans remain a prime focus. In a review of UNICEF publications from the years 1996 to 2010, Crivello and Chuta (2012) found that the number of publications tagged as "orphan" rose from 2 publications in 1996 to 610 in 2010. In George, the addition of vulnerability made few waves in services, which were already minimal, and mostly filled by nongovernmental organizations. For example, local workers who distributed resources to children identified dilemmas in serving OVCs because they did not have working definitions of vulnerability and most children fit some description of vulnerable because they lived in poverty. Parsing vulnerability presented so much of a challenge that fieldworkers continued streaming resources to children whose parent or parents had died.

CHAPTER 3 — BETWEEN SILENCE AND DISCLOSURE

1. Speaking publicly was also tied to material benefits from international organizations, including ARVs, in settings where people had few medical options to manage HIV (Nguyen 2010).

2. Issues of disclosure, and its benefits, are emphasized in a number of research articles, reports, and media accounts (Daniel et al. 2007; Family Health International 2003; Ishikawa et al. 2010; Kennedy et al. 2010; UNAIDS 2001).

3. See Durham and Klaits (2002) and Peters et al. (2008) on concealment. Other researchers have expressed ambivalence about the presumed "good" of disclosure (Bond 2010; Greeff et al. 2008). Liamputtong and Haritavorn's (2014) research with HIV positive women in Thailand led them to suggest that a woman's disclosure of her HIV to her children was not always positive. Also, see Carol Kidron's (2009) study of children of Holocaust survivors for a perspective on silence on topics that are not illness related.

4. Specifically, I draw on Kidron's (2009) ethnography of silence between Holocaust survivors and their children in which she talks about the silent presence of the Holocaust in material objects, facework, and mundane practices.

5. As part of the Zambia and South Africa Tuberculosis and AIDS Reduction Study (funded by the Gates Foundation), a team of researchers from ZAMBART conducted forty-six interviews with TB patients and twenty-one group discussions with elders, traditional healers, schoolchildren, and community-based health workers in George and other urban residential areas of Lusaka, Kitwe, Mansa, and Livingstone and in the rural setting of Pemba in Southern Province. The transcripts from these discussions and interviews were generously provided to me by ZAMBART. Quotes that come from the ZAMSTAR study are identified in endnotes. ZAMBART is not responsible for my interpretations; the analysis is my own.

6. ZAMSTAR focus group discussion with traditional healers in Maramba, June 4, 2005.

7. Ibid.

8. "Following the rules" refers to many things: listening to and respecting elders, adhering to customary practices, not engaging in excessive drinking and smoking, and following the advice of medical professionals and traditional healers. I discuss this phrase in more depth in chapter 4.

9. His reference to children is meant to indicate people older than the age of the children written about in this book.

10. ZAMSTAR focus group discussion with traditional healers in Maramba, June 4, 2005.

11. ZAMSTAR focus group discussion with community elders in Chimwemwe, July 13, 2005.

12. Ministry of Health (2005) lists this age range as the age range with the highest burden.

13. I noticed more children at the site of TB treatment in George in 2014 than I ever have before, which may be due to an increasing international and national push to get children tested and treated for TB and/or the real rise in active TB among children.

14. There are two exceptions: (1) vaccine campaigns and (2) the TB testing of children (usually aged six years) for latent TB to measure TB incidence in a population.

15. The World Health Organization, donors, and researchers increasingly acknowledge the need to focus on TB in children. However, even by 2014, there was little infrastructure to adequately diagnose and appropriately treat children in Zambia.

16. When someone dies in Zambia, people gather at their house or the house of a close relative, often spending several days and nights in close proximity to one another in mourning, prior to and after the burial.

17. Note the TB treatment supporter's slippage from TB to HIV here, which betrays the social reality in George that TB is often viewed as an underlying condition of HIV.

18. Quoted language from ZAMSTAR interviews.

19. I have discussed this particular finding in an article I published in the journal *AIDS Care* (Hunleth 2013a).

20. Bond and Nyblade (2006) demonstrated that clinical advice to avoid eating together during TB has led patients to express feelings of social isolation and abandonment.

21. See Moore and Vaughan (1994) on the importance of food sharing to social relationships in Zambia.

22. I risk simplifying the complexity of these claims and the historical, political, and economic contexts in which claims of the supernatural occur. There is a long literature on witchcraft and sorcery in Africa that does justice to the subject in ways that I cannot here. See, for example, Evans-Pritchard (1937). Adam Ashforth (2002, 2005) has written about witchcraft in the context of the AIDS epidemic in South Africa.

CHAPTER 4 — FOLLOWING THE MEDICINE

1. This chapter is a revised and expanded version of an article I published in *Medical Anthropology Quarterly* (Hunleth 2013b).

2. These are unregulated vehicles in varying states of disrepair that serve as a higher cost and private means of transportation in George. Buses provide the cheapest method

of transportation but there were no direct bus routes to the clinic during the years of my study.

3. For some examples of children as health and medicine promoters, see Ageel and Amin (1997), Bond et al. (2010), Foster et al. (2010), Guang-Han et al. (2005), and Onyango-Ouma et al. (2005).

4. See Biehl (2005) on pharmaceuticalization of healthcare, a process in which medication serves as medical care, particularly for people who are the most marginalized.

5. For more on the role of family in DOTS, see Frieden and Sbarbaro (2007) and Newell et al. (2006), among others.

6. Annual Report, "Republic of Zambia Ministry of Health Reports for the Year 1968."

7. Ibid.

8. Ibid., 29.

9. Personal communication with Virginia Bond on September 11, 2009. Bond interviewed Albert (a pseudonym).

10. Annual Report, "Republic of Zambia Ministry of Health Reports for the Years 1973–1977" and "Republic of Zambia Ministry of Health Reports for the Year 1978."

11. At this time, there was also a growing international recognition that the BCG vaccine was not sufficient for abating TB (Raviglione and Pio 2002).

12. This shortage and the growing concern over TB were reported in "Republic of Zambian Ministry of Health Reports" from both 1980 and 1983.

13. Behforouz, Farmer, and Mukherjee (2004) also discussed this shift from directly observed therapy to a more patient-centered model in their description of the use of community health promoters, who offered psychosocial support to patients on highly active antiretroviral therapy for HIV.

14. This renewal was probably prompted by donor demands.

15. TB Corners take varied and dynamic forms depending on health center architecture, populations served, and types of assistance given by NGOs.

16 The location of the TB Corner changed since I conducted my research. A new building was built behind the Breastfeeding building with support from an international NGO. See the final chapter in this book, "Childhood Tuberculosis."

17. Under the short-course regimen during 2007 and 2008, treatment lasted at least eight months and consisted of two phases: a two-month intensive phase and a six-month continuation phase. Concerns over the development of drug resistance to rifampicin, an active component in intensive phase treatment, meant that patients or family members were required to attend the TB Corner weekly during the intensive phase. They collected continuation phase medications monthly. While continuation phase was supposed to be a time when patients experience a return to health, such linear progression from sick to well did not occur for many people in my study, whose health declined when they stopped intensive treatment, due perhaps to HIV, poor living conditions, inadequate access to nutritious foods, and the removal of key medications in the continuation phase treatment.

18. I asked the children to identify all diseases that were pressing in George and then had them talk about each one of them in turn. See further explanation of this group discussion in chapter 3.

19. ZAMBART focus group discussion with traditional healers in George, May 5, 2005.

20. The pattern is the same across the surveys with most people recalling a positive reaction as encouragement to take medication.

21. Like Munyongo, Sarah also did not list her own children, whom she, too, believed were unaware of her diagnosis. However, later in the survey she said that the only people who cared for her during her illness were Tracy and her sons. See chapter 5.

22. Even though DOTS prescribes the sputum smear as the diagnostic test for detecting TB, Musonda was never offered a sputum test (to the best of my knowledge).

23. See Hansen's (1990) historical analysis of children in urban Zambia who provided labor to households without reciprocation or integration into the household.

CHAPTER 5 — CARE BY WOMEN AND CHILDREN

1. See chapter 4 for a description of the children's role play, in which Musa played the doctor. As the doctor, Musa made a judgment about the different care that mothers and aunts give to TB patients. It is hard to tell how much this resembled advice given to Musa's family when Patrick was ill. However, elements of the role play resonated with details of Patrick's illness and, just after Patrick's TB diagnosis, Musa's mother moved Patrick out of Nomsa's house.

2. See for example Evans-Pritchard (1937), Feierman (1985), Feierman and Janzen (1992), Janzen (1978), and Turner (1967, 1968).

3. See, for example, Biehl (2005) and Feierman (1985).

4. According to the World Health Organization (2015b), TB is one of the top five causes of death for women between the ages of fifteen and forty-four years.

5. Marxist-feminist researchers have described the household as a "locus of struggle" (Hartman 1981) and shown that we cannot talk about households as undifferentiated cooperative units. Rather, we should examine how gender, class, age, and other factors affect individual interests and roles.

6. Hansen's (1997) research in a different area of Lusaka showed that Sarah's experience, of not knowing how much her husband made or having access to his money, was more of the norm than exception.

7. Chitenge refers to a colorful fabric typically worn as a sarong or head wrapper by women in Zambia and other countries in East and southern Africa. Women also wear two-piece dresses, or suits, made from chitenge fabric.

8. See for example Bledsoe (1990), Colson (1958, 1971), and Shipton (2007).

9. Child rearing has been an important means through which women achieve social standing in Zambia and other places in Africa. See, as just a couple of examples, Bledsoe (2002) and Fortes (1969).

10. Unfortunately, we did not ask Sarah to answer these questions about Tracy, who had already moved out of the house.

11. Men took a different approach to the questions, and often emphasized their inability to provide food and clothing for the children.

12. I regularly looked through children's school notebooks to start conversations with them and because many children were proud of the work they did in school.

13. See Ross (2010) on the concept of accompaniment, particularly the imperative for community members to accompany the ill in settings of privation.

14. See Bury (1982) on the concept of biographical disruption during chronic illness.

Chapter 6 — Children and Global Health

1. See chapter 5.

2. See Introduction.

3. Parts of my assessment of child-oriented methodology in this chapter were previously published in *Childhood* (Hunleth 2011).

4. See Dorner 2015 on "ethics-post-practice" in research with children.

5. We published the results of the schoolchild intervention in the *International Journal of Tuberculosis and Lung Disease* (Bond et al. 2010).

6. To make this point, I have drawn on Alanen's (1988), Speier's (1976), and Thorne's (1987) critiques of theories of children's socialization.

7. See Janzen (1978) and Feierman (1985).

8. See Bluebond-Langner and Korbin (2007, 245) for a similar argument directed toward researchers of childhood in general.

9. Paul Farmer (1997, 1999) has written forcefully about the exaggeration of (adult) patient agency within the HIV epidemic, especially in the early years of the epidemic. Instead of focusing on broader political economic change or the policies that promoted the spread of HIV, interventions were focused instead on individual risk behaviors and the promotion of behavior change interventions.

10. See Farmer (1999, 9) for a critique of the uses of culture in commentaries on HIV and how culture hides the violence caused by political and economic processes.

11. These points follow Klaits's (2010) work in Botswana, in which he observes that love is an action that helps to nurture relationships, including relationships between the living and the dead.

Postscript: Childhood Tuberculosis

1. See Boulanger et al. (2016) for a review of ethical considerations in TB care in resource-poor settings. They cover issues such as the deprofessionalization of TB treatment, the risks health workers face in giving care, and the lack of compensation received by some treatment supporters.

References

Adams, Vincanne, Nancy J. Burke, and Ian Whitmarsh. 2014. "Slow Research: Thoughts for a Movement in Global Health." *Medical Anthropology* 33 (3): 179–197.

Ageel, A., and M. Amin. 1997. "Integration of Schistosomiasis-Control Activities into the Primary-Health-Care System in the Gizan Region, Saudi Arabia." *Annals of Tropical Medicine & Parasitology* 91 (8): 907–915.

Alanen, Leena. 1988. "Rethinking Childhood." *Acta Sociologica* 31 (1): 53–67.

Ansell, Nicola. 2016. "'Once Upon a Time . . .': Orphanhood, Childhood Studies and the Depoliticisation of Childhood Poverty in Southern Africa." *Childhood* 23 (2): 162–177.

Ansell, Nicola, and Lorraine van Blerk. 2004. "Children's Migration as a Household/Family Strategy: Coping with AIDS in Lesotho and Malawi." *Journal of Southern African Studies* 30 (3): 673–690.

Archambault, Caroline. 2010. "Fixing Families of Mobile Children: Recreating Kinship and Belonging among Maasai Adoptees in Kenya." *Childhood* 17 (2): 229–242.

Ariès, Philippe. 1962. *Centuries of Childhood: A Social History of Family Life*. London: Jonathan Cape Ltd.

Ashforth, Adam. 2002. "An Epidemic of Witchcraft? The Implications of AIDS for the Post-Apartheid State." *African Studies* 61 (1): 121–143.

———.2005. *Witchcraft, Violence, and Democracy in South Africa*. Chicago: University of Chicago Press.

Ayles, Helen, M. Muyoyeta, E. Du Toit, A. Schaap, S. Floyd, M. Simwinga, K. Shanaube, N. Chishinga, V. Bond, R. Dunbar, P. De Haas, A. James, N. C. Gey van Pittius, M. Claassens, K. Fielding, J. Fenty, C. Sismanidis, R. J. Hayes, N. Beyers, P. Godfrey-Faussett, and ZAMSTAR Team. 2013. "Effect of Household and Community Interventions on the Burden of Tuberculosis in Southern Africa: The ZAMSTAR Community-Randomised Trial." *Lancet* 382 (9899): 1183–1194.

Baron, David. 2010. "Zambia: Rationing Health by Queue." *PRI's The World*. Public Radio International. December 16, 2010. http://www.pri.org/stories/2010-12-16/rationing-health-series-part-3-zambia-rationing-health-queue.

Beall, Jo. 2002. "Globalization and Social Exclusion in Cities: Framing the Debate with Lessons from Africa and Asia." *Environment and Urbanization* 14 (1): 41–51.

Behforouz, Heidi L., Paul E. Farmer, and Joia S. Mukherjee. 2004. "From Directly Observed Therapy to Accompagnateurs: Enhancing AIDS Treatment Outcomes in Haiti and in Boston." *Clinical Infectious Diseases* 38 (Supplement 5): S429–S436.

Biehl, João. 2005. *Vita: Life in a Zone of Social Abandonment*. Berkeley: University of California Press.

Biehl, João, and Adriana Petryna. 2011. "Bodies of Rights and Therapeutic Markets." *Social Research* 78 (2): 359–394.

———. 2013a. "Critical Global Health." In *When People Come First: Critical Studies in Global Health*, edited by João Biehl and Adriana Petryna, 1–29. Princeton: Princeton University Press.

———, eds. 2013b. *When People Come First: Critical Studies in Global Health*. Princeton: Princeton University Press.

Bledsoe, Caroline. 1990. "'No Success without Struggle': Social Mobility and Hardship for Foster Children in Sierra Leone." *Man* 25 (1): 70–88.

———. 2002. *Contingent Lives: Fertility, Time, and Aging in West Africa*. Chicago: University of Chicago Press.

Bluebond-Langner, Myra. 1978. *The Private World of Dying Children*. Princeton: Princeton University Press.

Bluebond-Langner, Myra, and Jill Korbin. 2007. "Challenges and Opportunities in the Anthropology of Childhoods: An Introduction to 'Children, Childhoods, and Childhood Studies.'" *American Anthropologist* 109 (2): 241–246.

Bond, Virginia. 2010. "'It Is Not an Easy Decision on HIV, Especially in Zambia': Opting for Silence, Limited Disclosure, and Implicit Understanding to Retain a Wider Identity." *AIDS Care* 22 (Supplement 1): 6–13.

Bond, Virginia, Levi Chilikwela, Musonda Simwinga, Zenobe Reade, Helen Ayles, Peter Godfrey-Faussett, and Jean Hunleth. 2010. "Children's Role in Enhanced Case Finding in Zambia." *International Journal of Tuberculosis and Lung Disease* 14 (10): 1280–1287.

Bond, Virginia, and Laura Nyblade. 2006. "The Importance of Addressing the Unfolding TB-HIV Stigma in High HIV Prevalence Settings." *Journal of Community & Applied Social Psychology* 16 (6): 452–461.

Bosman, M. C. 2000. "Health Sector Reform and Tuberculosis Control: The Case of Zambia." *International Journal of Tuberculosis and Lung Disease* 4 (7): 606–614.

Boulanger, Renaud F., Matthew R. Hunt, and Solomon R. Benatar. 2016. "Where Caring Is Sharing: Evolving Ethical Considerations in Tuberculosis Prevention among Healthcare Workers." *Clinical Infectious Diseases* 62 (Supplement 3): S268–S274.

Bray, Rachel. 2003. "Who Does the Housework? An Examination of South African Children's Working Roles." *Social Dynamics* 29 (2): 95–131.

———. 2009. "How Does AIDS Illness Affect Women's Residential Decisions? Findings from an Ethnographic Study in a Cape Town Township." *African Journal of AIDS Research* 8 (2): 167–179.

Bray, Rachel, and René Brandt. 2007. "Child Care and Poverty in South Africa: An Ethnographic Challenge to Conventional Interpretations." *Journal of Children & Poverty* 13 (1): 1–19.

Buch, Elana. 2015. "Anthropology of Aging and Care." *Annual Review of Anthropology* 44 (1): 277–293.

Bury, Michael. 1982. "Chronic Illness as Biographical Disruption." *Sociology of Health and Illness* 4 (2): 167–182.

Chawla, Louise. 2002. "Toward Better Cities for Children and Youth." In *Growing Up in an Urbanising World*, edited by Louise Chawla, 219–240. New York: Earthscan.

Cheney, Kristen. 2007. *Pillars of the Nation: Child Citizens and Ugandan National Development*. Chicago: University of Chicago Press.

Chintu, Victor, Victor Mudenda, Sebastian Lucas, Andrew Nunn, Kennedy Lishimpi, Daniel Maswahu, Francis Kasoko, Peter Mwaba, Ganapati Bhat, and Alimuddin Terunuma. 2002. "Lung Diseases at Necropsy in African Children Dying from Respiratory Illnesses: A Descriptive Necropsy Study." *Lancet* 360 (9338): 986–990.

Cliggett, Lisa, and Brooke Wyssmann. 2009. "Crimes against the Future: Zambian Teachers' Alternative Income Generation and the Undermining of Education." *Africa Today* 55 (3): 25–43.

Cole, Jennifer, and Deborah Durham, eds. 2007. *Generations and Globalization: Youth, Age, and Family in the New World Economy*. Bloomington: Indiana University Press.

Colson, Elizabeth. 1958. *Marriage and the Family among the Plateau Tonga of Northern Rhodesia*. Manchester: Manchester University Press.

———. 1971. *Kariba Studies IV: The Social Consequences of Resettlement*. Manchester: Manchester University Press.

Crehan, Kate. 1997. "Of Chickens and Guinea Fowl: Living Matriliny in North-Western Zambia in the 1980s." *Critique of Anthropology* 17 (2): 211–227.

Crivello, Gina, and Nardos Chuta. 2012. "Rethinking Orphanhood and Vulnerability in Ethiopia." *Development in Practice* 22 (4): 536–548.

Daniel, Marguerite, Hellen Malinga Apila, Rune Bjorgo, and Gro Therese Lie. 2007. "Breaching Cultural Silence: Enhancing Resilience among Ugandan Orphans." *African Journal of AIDS Research* 6 (2): 109–120.

Dorner, Lisa M. 2015. "From Relating to (Re)Presenting: Challenges and Lessons Learned from an Ethnographic Study with Young Children." *Qualitative Inquiry* 21 (4): 354–365.

Durham, Deborah, and Frederick Klaits. 2002. "Funerals and the Public Space of Sentiment in Botswana." *Journal of Southern African Studies* 28 (4): 773–791.

Edwards, Rosalind, and Pam Alldred. 1999. "Children and Young People's Views of Social Research: The Case of Research on Home-School Relations." *Childhood* 6 (2): 261–281.

Emerson, Robert M., Rachel I. Fretz, and Linda L. Shaw. 1995. *Writing Ethnographic Fieldnotes*. Chicago: University of Chicago Press.

Evans, Ruth, and Saul Becker. 2009. *Children Caring for Parents with HIV and AIDS: Global Issues and Policy Responses*. Chicago: University of Chicago Press.

Evans-Pritchard, E. E. [1937] 1976. *Witchcraft, Oracles, and Magic among the Azande*. New York: Oxford University Press.

Family Health International. 2003. *Voices from the Community: The Impact of HIV/AIDS on the Lives of Orphaned Children and Their Guardians*. Bloomington: Family Health International.

Farmer, Paul. 1997. "Social Scientists and the New Tuberculosis." *Social Science & Medicine* 44 (3): 347–358.

———. 1999. *Infections and Inequalities: The Modern Plague*. Berkeley: University of California Press.

———. 2013. "Preface." In *Reimagining Global Health*, edited by Paul Farmer, Jim Yong Kim, Arthur Kleinman, and Matthew Basilico, 111–132. Berkeley: University of California Press.

Farmer, Paul, Jim Yong Kim, Arthur Kleinman, and Matthew Basilico, eds. 2013. *Reimagining Global Health: An Introduction*. Berkeley: University of California Press.

Fassin, Didier. 2013. "Children as Victims: The Moral Economy of Childhood in the Time of AIDS." In *When People Come First: Critical Studies in Global Health*, edited by João Biehl and Adriana Petryna, 109–129. Princeton: Princeton University Press.

Feierman, Steven. 1985. "Struggles for Control: The Social Roots of Health and Healing in Modern Africa." *African Studies Review* 28 (2/3): 73–147.

Feierman, Steven, and John M. Janzen. 1992. *The Social Basis of Health and Healing in Africa.* Berkeley: University of California Press.

Ferguson, James. 1999. *Expectations of Modernity: Myths and Meanings of Urban Life on the Zambian Copperbelt.* Berkeley: University of California Press.

Fortes, Meyer. 1969. *Kinship and the Social Order: The Legacy of L. H. Morgan.* Chicago: Aldine Publishing Company.

Foster, S. D., S. Nakamanya, R. Kyomuhangi, J. Amurwon, G. Namara, B. Amuron, C. Nabiryo, J. Birungi, B. Wolff, S. Jaffar, and H. Grosskurth. 2010. "The Experience of 'Medicine Companions' to Support Adherence to Antiretroviral Therapy: Quantitative and Qualitative Data from a Trial Population in Uganda." *AIDS Care* 22 (Supplement 1): 35–43.

Frieden, Thomas, and John Sbarbaro. 2007. "Promoting Adherence to Treatment for Tuberculosis: The Importance of Direct Observation." *Bulletin of the World Health Organization* 85 (5): 407–409.

Gallacher, Lesley-Anne, and Michael Gallagher. 2008. "Methodological Immaturity in Childhood Research? Thinking through 'Participatory Methods.'" *Childhood* 15 (4): 499–516.

Garcia, Angela. 2010. *The Pastoral Clinic: Addiction and Dispossession along the Rio Grande.* Berkeley: University of California Press.

Global Fund. 2016. *The Global Fund Overview.* The Global Fund to Fight AIDS, Tuberculosis, and Malaria. Accessed February 20, 2016. http://www.theglobalfund.org/en/overview/.

Gonzalez de la Rocha, Mercedes. 2007. "The Construction of the Myth of Survival." *Development and Change* 38 (1): 45–66.

Good, Mary Jo Del-Vecchio. 2001. "The Biotechnical Embrace." *Culture, Medicine, and Psychiatry* 25 (4): 395–410.

Greeff, Minrie, Rene Phetlhu, Lucia N. Makoae, Priscilla S. Dlamini, William L. Holzemer, Joanne R. Naidoo, Thecia W. Kohi, Leana R. Uys, and Maureen L. Chirwa. 2008. "Disclosure of HIV Status: Experiences and Perceptions of Persons Living with HIV/AIDS and Nurses Involved in Their Care in Africa." *Qualitative Health Research* 18 (3): 311–324.

Guang-Han, Hu, Hu Jia, Song Kuang-Yu, Lin Dan-Dan, Zhang Ju, Cao Chun-Li, Xu Jing, Li Dong, and Jiang We-Seng. 2005. "The Role of Health Education and Health Promotion in the Control of Schistosomiasis: Experiences from a 12-Year Intervention Study in the Poyang Lake Area." *Acta Tropica* 96 (2/3): 232–241.

Hansen, Karen Tranberg. 1990. "Labor Migration and Urban Child Labor during the Colonial Period in Zambia." In *Demography from Scanty Evidence*, edited by Bruce Fetter, 219–234. Boulder, CO: Lynne Rienner Publishers.

———. 1997. *Keeping House in Lusaka.* New York: Columbia University Press.

———. 2005. "Getting Stuck in the Compound: Some Odds against Social Adulthood in Lusaka, Zambia." *Africa Today* 51 (4): 3–16.

Hardman, Charlotte. 1973. "Can There Be an Anthropology of Children?" *Journal of the Anthropological Society of Oxford* 4 (2): 85–99.

Harper, Ian. 2006. "Anthropology, DOTS, and Understanding Tuberculosis Control in Nepal." *Journal of Biosocial Science* 38 (1): 57–67.

———. 2010. "Extreme Condition, Extreme Measures? Compliance, Drug Resistance, and the Control of Tuberculosis." *Anthropology & Medicine* 17 (2): 201–214.

Hartmann, Heidi. 1981. "The Family as the Locus of Gender, Class, and Political Struggle: The Example of Housework." *Signs* 6 (3): 366–394.

Hecht, Tobias. 1998. *At Home in the Street: Street Children of Northeast Brazil*. Cambridge: Cambridge University Press.

Henderson, Patricia. 2013. "AIDS, Metaphor, and Ritual: The Crafting of Care in Rural South African Childhoods." *Childhood* 20 (1): 9–21.

Henneken, Charles H., and Julie E. Buring. 1987. *Epidemiology in Medicine*. Boston: Little, Brown and Company.

Hochschild, Arlie Russell. 2003. *The Managed Heart: Commercialization of Human Feeling*. Berkeley: University of California Press.

Hunleth, Jean. 2011. "Beyond *On* or *With*: Questioning Power Dynamics and Knowledge Production in 'Child-Oriented' Research Methodology." *Childhood* 18 (1): 81–93.

———. 2013a. "'ARVs' as Sickness and Medicine: Examining Children's Knowledge and Experience in the HIV Era in Urban Zambia." *AIDS Care* 25 (6): 763–766.

———. 2013b. "Children's Roles in Tuberculosis Treatment Regimes: Constructing Childhood and Kinship in Urban Zambia." *Medical Anthropology Quarterly* 27 (2): 292–311.

Hunleth, Jean, Rebekah Jacob, Steven Cole, Virginia Bond, and Aimee James. 2015. "School Holidays: Examining Childhood, Gender Norms, and Kinship in Children's Shorter-Term Residential Mobility in Zambia." *Children's Geographies* 13 (5): 501–517.

Ishikawa, Naoko, Pat Pridmore, Roy Carr-Hill, and Kreangkrai Chaimuangdee. 2010. "Breaking Down the Wall of Silence around Children Affected by AIDS in Thailand to Support Their Psychosocial Health." *AIDS Care* 22 (3): 308–313.

James, Allison, and Adrian James. 2012. *Key Concepts in Childhood Studies*. 2nd ed. Los Angeles: Sage.

Janzen, John M. 1978. *The Quest for Therapy in Lower Zaire*. Berkeley: University of California Press.

JICA. 2004. "Water Supply Project in Satellite Area of Lusaka, George Community Empowerment Program, and Lusaka District Primary Health Care (PHC) Project." *Achieving More Effective Cooperation: Annual Evaluation Report 2004*. Accessed February 14, 2016. http://www.jica.go.jp/english/our_work/evaluation/reports/2004/pdf/2004_03.pdf.

Kaona, Frederick, Mary Tuba, Seter Siziya, and Lenganji Sikaona. 2004. "An Assessment of Factors Contributing to Treatment Adherence and Knowledge of TB Transmission among Patients on TB Treatment." *BMC Public Health* 4: 68.

Kapata, Nathan, Pascalina Chanda-Kapata, Justin O'Grady, Matthew Bates, Peter Mwaba, Saskia Janssen, Ben Marais, Frank Cobelens, Martin Grobusch, and Alimuddin Zumla. 2013. "Trends in Childhood Tuberculosis in Zambia: A Situation Analysis." *Journal of Tropical Pediatrics* 59 (2): 134–139.

Kelly, Michael J. 2008. "Adult Literacy Globally and in Zambia." *Jesuit Center for Theological Reflection Bulletin*. Accessed June 19, 2009. http://www.jctr.org.zm/14-jctr-bulletin/40-jctr-bulletin.

Kennedy, David P., Burton O. Cowgill, Laura M. Bogart, Rosalie Corona, Gery W. Ryan, Debra A. Murphy, Theresa Nguyen, and Mark A. Schuster. 2010. "Parents' Disclosure of Their HIV Infection to Their Children in the Context of the Family." *AIDS Behavior* 14 (5): 1095–1105.

Kidron, Carol A. 2009. "Toward an Ethnography of Silence: The Lived Presence of the Past in the Everyday Life of Holocaust Trauma Survivors and Their Descendants in Israel." *Current Anthropology* 50 (1): 5–26.

Klaits, Frederick. 2010. *Death in a Church of Life: Moral Passion during Botswana's Time of AIDS.* Berkeley: University of California Press.

Koch, Erin. 2006. "Valuing Life, Weighing Death: Beyond Suspicion: Evidence, (Un)Certainty, and Tuberculosis in Georgian Prisons." *American Ethnologist* 33 (1): 50–62.

———. 2013. *Free Market Tuberculosis: Managing Epidemics in Post-Soviet Georgia.* Nashville: Vanderbilt University Press.

Lancaster, Chet S. 1981. *The Goba of Zambia: Sex, Roles, Economics, and Change.* Norman: University of Oklahoma Press.

Langevang, Thilde, and Katherine V. Gough. 2009. "Surviving through Moving: The Mobility of Urban Youth in Ghana." *Social & Cultural Geography* 10 (7): 741–756.

Leinhardt, Christian, and Jessica Ogden. 2004. "Tuberculosis Control in Resource-Poor Countries: Have We Reached the Limits of the Universal Paradigm?" *Tropical Medicine and International Health* 9 (7): 833–841.

Liamputtong, Pranee, and Niphattra Haritavorn. 2014. "To Tell or Not to Tell: Disclosure to Children and Family amongst Thai Women Living with HIV/AIDS." *Health Promotion International.* Published online July 17, 2014.

Livingston, Julie. 2005. *Debility and the Moral Imagination in Botswana.* Bloomington: Indiana University Press.

———. 2012. *Improvising Medicine: An African Oncology Ward in an Emerging Cancer Epidemic.* Durham, NC: Duke University Press.

Madison, Soyini. 2012. *Critical Ethnography: Method, Ethics, and Performance.* 2nd ed. Los Angeles: Sage.

Meintjes, Helen, and Sonja Geise. 2006. "Spinning the Epidemic: The Making of Mythologies of Orphanhood in the Context of AIDS." *Childhood* 13 (3): 407–430.

Messac, Luke, and Krishna Prabhu. 2013. "Redefining the Possible." In *Reimagining Global Health,* edited by Paul Farmer, Jim Yong Kim, Arthur Kleinman, and Matthew Basilico, 111–132. Berkeley: University of California Press.

Ministry of Education. 2006. "Millennium Development Goals Status Report 2005." Lusaka: Ministry of Education.

———. 2010. "Free Education in Zambia: Most Frequently Asked Questions on Free Education." Lusaka: Ministry of Education.

Ministry of Health. 2005. "National Health Strategic Plan 2006–2010." Lusaka: Ministry of Health.

Moore, Henrietta. 1994. *A Passion for Difference: Essays in Anthropology and Gender.* Bloomington: Indiana University Press.

Moore, Henrietta, and Megan Vaughan. 1994. *Cutting Down Trees: Gender, Nutrition, and Change in the Northern Province of Zambia, 1890–1990.* New York: Heinemann.

Morgan, Myfanwy, Sara Gibbs, Krista Maxwell, and Nicky Britten. 2002. "Hearing Children's Voices: Methodological Issues in Conducting Focus Groups with Children Aged 7–11 Years." *Qualitative Research* 2 (1): 5–20.

Mulenga, Chanda, David Mwakazanga, Kim Vereecken, Shepherd Khondowe, Nathan Kapata, Isdore Chola Shamputa, Heman Meulemans, and Leen Rigouts. 2010. "Management of Pulmonary Tuberculosis Patients in an Urban Setting in Zambia: A Patient's Perspective." *BMC Public Health* 10: 756.

Muzenda-Mudavanhu, Chipo. 2016. "A Review of Children's Participation in Disaster Risk Reduction." *Jàmbá: Journal of Disaster Risk Studies* 8 (1).

Mwaba, P., M. Maboshe, C. Chintu, B. Squire, S. Nyirenda, R. Sunkutu, and A. Zumla. 2003. "The Relentless Spread of Tuberculosis in Zambia—Trends over the Past 37 Years (1964–2000)." *South African Medical Journal* 93 (2): 149–152.

Mweemba, P., C. Haruzivishe, S. Siziya, P. J. Chipimo, K. Cristenson, and E. Johansson. 2008. "Knowledge, Attitude and Compliance with Tuberculosis Treatment, Lusaka, Zambia." *Medical Journal of Zambia* 35 (4): 121–128.

Newell, James, Sushl Baral, Shanta Pande, Dirgh Bam, and Pushpa Maiia. 2006. "Family-Member DOTS and Community DOTS for Tuberculosis Control in Nepal: Cluster-Randomised Controlled Trial." *Lancet* 367 (9514): 903–909.

Nguyen, Vinh-Kim. 2005. "Antiretroviral Globalism, Biopolitics, and Therapeutic Citizenship." In *Global Assemblages: Technology, Politics, and Ethics as Anthropological Problems*, edited by Aihwa Ong and Stephen Collier, 124–144. Malden, MA: Blackwell Publishing.

———. 2010. *The Republic of Therapy: Triage and Sovereignty in West Africa's Time of AIDS*. Durham, NC: Duke University Press.

Ngwane, Zolani. 2003. "'Christmas Time' and the Struggles for the Household in the Countryside: Rethinking the Cultural Geography of Migrant Labour in South Africa." *Journal of Southern African Studies* 29 (3): 681–699.

Notermans, Catrien. 2008. "The Emotional World of Kinship: Children's Experiences of Fosterage in East Cameroon." *Childhood* 15 (3): 355–377.

Office for National Statistics. 2013. "Providing Unpaid Care May Have an Adverse Effect on Young Carers' General Health." In *2011 Census Detailed Characteristics for Local Authorities in England and Wales*. United Kingdom: Office for National Statistics.

Onyango-Ouma, W., J. Aagaard-Hansen, and B. B. Jensen. 2005. "The Potential of School-children as Health Change Agents in Rural Western Kenya." *Social Science & Medicine* 61 (8): 1711–1722.

Orellana, Marjorie Faulstich. 2009. *Translating Childhoods: Immigrant Youth, Language, and Culture*. New Brunswick, NJ: Rutgers University Press.

Percy-Smith, Barry. 2002. "Contested Worlds: Constraints and Opportunities in City and Suburban Environments in an English Midlands City." In *Growing Up in an Urbanising World*, edited by Louise Chawla, 57–80. New York: Earthscan.

Peters, Pauline E., Peter A. Walker, and Daimon Kambewa. 2008. "Striving for Normality in a Time of AIDS in Malawi." *Journal of Modern African Studies* 46 (4): 659–687.

Petryna, Adriana. 2002. *Life Exposed: Biological Citizens after Chernobyl*. Princeton: Princeton University Press.

Pfeiffer, James. 2013. "The Struggle for a Public Sector: PEPFAR in Mozambique." In *When People Come First: Critical Studies in Global Health*, edited by João Biehl and Adriana Petryna, 166–181. Princeton: Princeton University Press.

Pigg, Stacy Leigh. 2013. "On Sitting and Doing: Ethnography as Action in Global Health." *Social Science & Medicine* 99: 127–134.

Rakner, Lise. 2003. *Political and Economic Liberalisation in Zambia 1991–2001*. Stockholm: Elanders Gotab.

Raviglione, M. C., and A. Pio. 2002. "Evolution of WHO Policies for Tuberculosis Control, 1948–2001." *Lancet* 359 (9308): 775–780.

Reynolds, Pamela. 1991. *Dance Civet Cat: Child Labour in the Zambezi Valley*. Athens: Ohio University Press.

Richards, M. 1969. "Tuberculosis." *Zambia Nursing Journal* 3 (4): 19–22.

Rohr-Rouendaal, Petra. 1997. *Where There Is No Artist: Development Drawings and How to Use Them.* London: Intermediate Technology Publications.

Rose, Nikolas, and Carlos Novas. 2005. "Biological Citizenship." In *Global Assemblages: Technology, Politics, and Ethics as Anthropological Problems*, edited by Aihwa Ong and Stephen Collier, 439–463. Oxford: Blackwell.

Ross, Fiona. 2010. *Raw Life, New Hope: Decency, Housing and Everyday Life in a Post-Apartheid Community.* Cape Town, South Africa: UCT Press.

Schlyter, Ann. 1984. *Upgrading Reconsidered: The George Studies in Retrospect.* Gävle: National Swedish Institute for Building Research.

———. 2009. "Body Politics and the Crafting of Citizenship in Peri-Urban Lusaka." *Feminist Africa* 13: 23–43.

Schlyter, Ann, and Thomas Schlyter. 1979. *George: The Development of a Squatter Settlement in Lusaka, Zambia.* Stockholm: Swedish Council for Building Research.

Schwartzman, Helen. 1978. *Transformations: The Anthropology of Children's Play.* New York: Plenum Press.

Shin, Sonya, Jennifer Furin, Jaime Bayona, Kedar Mate, Jim Yong Kim, and Paul Farmer. 2004. "Community-Based Treatment of Multidrug-Resistant Tuberculosis in Lima, Peru: Seven Years of Experience." *Social Science and Medicine* 59 (7): 1529–1539.

Shipton, Parker. 2007. *The Nature of Entrustment: Intimacy, Exchange, and the Sacred in Africa.* New Haven: Yale University Press.

Skovdal, Morten, and Vincent Ogutu. 2009. "'I Washed and Fed My Mother before Going to School': Understanding the Psychosocial Well-Being of Children Providing Chronic Care for Adults Affected by HIV/AIDS in Western Kenya." *Global Health* 5 (8).

Speier, Matthew. 1976. "The Adult Ideological Viewpoint in Studies of Childhood." In *Rethinking Childhood: Perspectives on Development and Society*, edited by Arlene Skolnick, 168–186. Boston: Little, Brown and Company.

Spitulnik, Debra. 1998. "The Language of the City: Town Bemba as Urban Hybridity." *Journal of Linguistic Anthropology* 8 (1): 30–59.

Stack, Carol. 1974. *All Our Kin.* New York: BasicBooks.

Swart-Kruger, Jill. 2002. "Children in a South African Squatter Camp Gain and Lose a Voice." In *Growing Up in an Urbanising World*, edited by Louise Chawla, 111–133. New York: Earthscan.

Thorne, Barrie. 1987. "Re-visioning Women and Social Change: Where Are the Children?" *Gender & Society* 1 (1): 85–109.

———. 1993. *Gender Play: Girls and Boys in School.* New Brunswick, NJ: Rutgers University Press.

Toren, Christina. 2007. "Sunday Lunch in Fiji: Continuity and Transformation in Ideas of the Household." *American Anthropologist* 109 (2): 285–295.

Turner, Victor. 1967. *Forest of Symbols.* Ithaca, NY: Cornell University Press.

———. 1968. *Drums of Affliction.* Oxford: Oxford University Press.

UNAIDS. 2001. "Investing in Our Future: Psychosocial Support for Children Affected by HIV/AIDS: A Case Study in Zimbabwe and the United Republic of Tanzania." In *UNAIDS Best Practice Collection.* Geneva: UNAIDS.

———. 2014. *Zambia: HIV and AIDS Estimates (2014).* Accessed February 20, 2016. http://www.unaids.org/en/regionscountries/countries/zambia.

Ungruhe, Christian. 2010. "Symbols of Success: Youth, Peer Pressure, and the Role of Adulthood among Juvenile Male Return Migrants in Ghana." *Childhood* 17 (2): 259–271.

UNICEF. 2004. *Orphans and Vulnerable Children in Zambia 2004 Situation Analysis*. Lusaka: Ministry of Sport, Youth, and Child Development.

———. 2008. *Zambia: Situation Analysis of Children and Women 2008*. Lusaka: UNICEF Zambia.

———. 2016. "Zambia: Statistics." Accessed July 22, 2016. http://www.unicef.org/infoby-country/zambia_statistics.html.

UNOPS. 2015. "Stop TB Partnership Annual Report 2014." Geneva: UNOPS.

Whyte, Susan Reynolds. 2014a. "Introduction: The First Generation." In *Second Chances: Surviving AIDS in Uganda*, edited by Susan Reynolds Whyte, 1–24. Durham, NC: Duke University Press.

———, ed. 2014b. *Second Chances: Surviving AIDS in Uganda*. Durham, NC: Duke University Press.

Whyte, Susan Reynolds, Hanne O. Mogensen, and Jenipher Twebaze. 2014. "Families." In *Second Chances: Surviving AIDS in Uganda*, edited by Susan Reynolds Whyte, 104–117. Durham, NC: Duke University Press.

World Bank. 2002. "Upgrading of Low Income Settlements: Country Assessment Report: Zambia." Accessed February 20, 2016.http://siteresources.worldbank.org/INTUSU/Resources/zambia.pdf.

World Health Organization. 1994. "WHO Tuberculosis Programme: Framework for Effective Tuberculosis Control." Geneva: World Health Organization.

———. 1997. "Anti-Tuberculosis Drug Resistance in the World." In *The WHO/IUATLD Global Project on Anti-tuberculosis Drug Resistance Surveillance 1994–1997*. Geneva: World Health Organization.

———. 2003. "Community Contribution to TB Care: Practice and Policy: Review of Experience of Community Contribution to TB Care and Recommendations to National TB Programmes." Geneva: World Health Organization.

———. 2013. "Roadmap for Childhood Tuberculosis: Towards Zero Deaths." Geneva: World Health Organization.

———. 2015a. "Tuberculosis Country Profiles: Zambia." Geneva: World Health Organization.

———. 2015b. "Tuberculosis: Key Facts." Accessed February 20, 2016. http://www.who.int/mediacentre/factsheets/fs104/en/.

Young, Lorraine. 2003. "The 'Place' of Street Children in Kampala, Uganda: Marginalisation, Resistance, and Acceptance in the Urban Environment." *Environment and Planning D: Society and Space* 21 (5): 607–627.

ZAMBART. 2011. "Press Statement for Immediate Release: Levels of MDR TB Are Low in Zambia According to New Survey." Accessed May 6, 2012. http://www.zambart.org/wp-content/uploads/press_release_040311_drs_final.pdf.

Index

Page references with an f indicate a figure.

About the Author

Jean Hunleth has worked on issues related to health and infectious disease in Zambia since 1999, when she first lived in rural Eastern Province, Zambia, as a Peace Corps volunteer. Hunleth's published works focus on children's caregiving roles, children's participation in healthcare programming, research methods for working with children in adversity, and the lived experience of healthcare inequalities in the United States and Zambia. She is a former Fulbright fellow and has received funding for her research and training from the National Science Foundation, the Wenner-Gren Foundation for Anthropological Research, the American Association of University Women (AAUW), and the National Institutes of Health. Hunleth holds a doctorate degree in cultural anthropology and a master's degree in public health from Northwestern University and received postdoctoral training in community-based cancer research at Washington University in St. Louis. She is currently a research scientist in the Division of Public Health Sciences at Washington University in St. Louis.

Available titles in the Rutgers Series in Childhood Studies

CPSIA information can be obtained
at www.ICGtesting.com
Printed in the USA
LVHW04s2003181018
594071LV00001B/19/P